*Heart Illness
and Intimacy*

Heart Illness and Intimacy

How Caring Relationships Aid Recovery

. . . . . .

WAYNE M. SOTILE, Ph.D.

The Johns Hopkins University Press

BALTIMORE AND LONDON

The Johns Hopkins University Press
701 West 40th Street
Baltimore, Maryland 21211-2190
The Johns Hopkins Press Ltd., London

This book is not intended to provide medical or legal advice.
The services of a competent professional should be obtained
whenever medical, legal, or other specific advice is needed.

The paper used in this book meets the minimum
requirements of American National Standard for
Information Sciences—Permanence of Paper
for Printed Library Materials, ANSI Z39.48-1984.

Library of Congress Cataloging-in-Publication Data

Sotile, Wayne M., 1951–
Heart illness and intimacy : how caring relationships aid recovery /
Wayne M. Sotile.
p.   cm.
Includes bibliographical references and index.
ISBN 0-8018-4290-5 (alk. paper)
1. Heart—Diseases—Patients—Family relationships. 2. Heart—
Diseases—Patients—Rehabilitation.   I. Title. [DNLM:
1. Adaptation, Psychological. 2. Family—psychology. 3. Heart
Disease—rehabilitation. 4. Marriage.   WG 200 S717h]
RC682.S64   1992
616.1'2'0019—dc20
DNLM/DLC for Library of Congress   91-20831

To Mary—
my wife, best friend, editor, and colleague
and only partner—

and

To my daughters, Rebecca and Julia,
for being so impressed that I could write a book,
for being so impressed with me whether
I write books or not,
and—most of all—just for being.

I love you all with my life.

Contents

■ ■ ■ ■ ■ ■

Foreword, by Henry S. Miller, Jr., M.D.   ix

Acknowledgments   xiii

Introduction   xv

Part I The Family as a Team in Sickness and in Health

1. A Family in Distress   3
2. The Many Stresses of Illness   8
3. Family Teams   12
4. Healthy Family Reactions to Illness   21
5. Pitfalls of Family Life   40
6. Adult Children of Heart Patients   60

Part II Intimacy: The Key to Health

7. Pictures of a Healthy Marriage   77
8. Sex and Heart Illness   100

Part III The Personality Factor: Can We Change?

9. Personality   141
10. Marriage and Type A Personalities   160

11. *Living with Type A's*   *183*

12. *Strategies for Changing Type A Patterns*   *202*

Part IV More Than Surviving: Thriving

13. *Helping Each Other by Helping Yourself*   *219*

14. *The Importance of Attitude*   *237*

15. *Healing*   *248*

Appendix A: Resources   *259*

Appendix B: Choosing a Therapist   *263*

Recommended Reading   *267*

References   *271*

Index   *285*

Foreword

∎ ∎ ∎ ∎ ∎ ∎

Heart disease, stroke, hypertension, and vascular disease account for more than 55 percent of all medical problems in the United States. Even though the mortality from these problems has decreased by more than 30 percent in the past twenty years, these health problems still occur more frequently than all other illnesses combined.

As therapy has been improved and mortality reduced, the need for sophisticated rehabilitation and long-term care strategies has become greater. Accordingly, it has become increasingly evident that the evaluation and treatment of psychological problems experienced by heart patients are as important to rehabilitation as is control of cardiovascular symptoms, diet, blood pressure, and other risk factors.

We are only now beginning to recognize the extent to which heart illness affects families—not just patients. The threatened loss of a husband, wife, father, mother, breadwinner, lover, or educator can be devastating to families. Unfortunately, very little has been written regarding this important topic until now.

Wayne Sotile, Ph.D., is a member of the first wave of a relatively new group of professionals who have been added to cardiac rehabilitation teams. Being painfully aware of the various psychological, behavioral and family problems that have long plagued heart patients—but also being unable to evaluate accurately and provide adequate therapy

for these patients—cardiac rehabilitation teams have turned to psychologists and psychiatrists for help.

The addition of experts like Dr. Sotile to our cardiac rehabilitation
teams has proven to be of immeasurable assistance to practicing cardiologists, internists, family physicians, and cardiovascular surgeons.
Mental health professionals have educated physicians, patients, and
families about effective ways to control the psychological factors affecting cardiac rehabilitation. The benefit of such information has become evident in cardiac rehabilitation. With such help, we have l een
able to maximize recovery from heart illness and facilitate patients'
return to work and resumption of viable roles in their families.

Dr. Sotile has directed the psychological team in our cardiac rehabilitation program for the past thirteen years. His experience with patient therapy and family counseling for patients suffering from a wide
range of medical problems has provided him with the expertise and
experience ideally suited to the team. His abilities to pursue and detect
the patient's real problems and to incorporate the rehabilitation staff
and community resources into the treatment of these stressors have
made him unique in the field. His lectures to patients, families, and
staff have been highlights in our program. His very descriptive comments during patient evaluation meetings with our staff—always delivered with his unique blend of Louisiana and Italian humor—have
made him maximally effective.

In this book, Dr. Sotile's wealth of knowledge and experience
shine forth. He opens with an extensive case history of a family whose
reactions are used throughout the early chapters as pointed examples
of various important problems faced by heart patients and their families. Chapter 2 explains how living with heart illness involves coping
with multiple stressors for both patient and family. In chapters 3, 4,
and 5 he realistically explains how families work and how marriage
and family problems experienced during everyday living can be affected by heart disease. His emphasis on both healthy and unhealthy
family reactions to illness provides helpful points of comparison. In
chapter 6, his descriptions of problems faced by adult children of heart
patients are particularly relevant and will be useful to any family coping with the chronic illness of a parent.

In chapters 7 and 8, the expertise, compassion, and humor that are hallmarks of Dr. Sotile's uniquely effective style of helping couples to improve their marriages become obvious. His descriptions of specific tools that any couple can use to better their marriage are concise and down-to-earth. His summary of the wealth of information available on sexual aspects of cardiac rehabilitation is perhaps this book's most shining point of excellence. Chapters 9 through 12 provide an extensive discussion of the important topic of how personality affects reactions to heart illness. Once again, with clarity and multiple case examples drawn from his own extensive experience, Dr. Sotile thoroughly explores the behavior of Type A personalities and the rehabilitation tasks they and their spouses face.

Dr. Sotile concludes with three chapters that provide invaluable guidelines to anyone who wants to learn how to manage stress better during highly emotional times. His final chapter, "Healing," will stir in any couple a spirit of loving concern for each other. Throughout the book, Dr. Sotile expertly integrates information from more than two hundred carefully selected references and from his vast clinical experience. His case examples bring his material alive and lend a lasting ring of truth to the points being made.

Dr. Sotile has written a book that will make a major contribution to the literature. It will be of lasting benefit to heart patients and their families and to medical practitioners treating heart and vascular diseases. In keeping with his personal style, Dr. Sotile has kept his comments short and to the point, even though a wealth of information is presented. This book will be an excellent source of information for anyone interested in better understanding patient and family reactions to any illness and specifically to cardiovascular disease.

In this publication, Dr. Sotile shares with the public the knowledge and effective therapeutic techniques that we medical professionals have long been exclusively privileged to apply in our cardiac rehabilitation programs and medical practices. We are happy to share him with you. Read on, and enjoy.

Henry S. Miller, Jr., M.D.

Henry S. Miller, Jr., M.D., is professor of medicine and cardiology at the Bowman Gray School of Medicine, Wake Forest University, and medical director of the Wake Forest University Cardiac Rehabilitation Program. He is a past president of the American College of Sports Medicine.

Acknowledgments

∎ ∎ ∎ ∎ ∎

Many people have encouraged, coached, and supported me as I have written this book. I offer my sincere thanks and appreciation to:

Henry Miller, M.D., and Paul Ribisl, Ph.D., for introducing me to the field of cardiac rehabilitation, for their support and help in publicizing this project, for their endorsement of my work and of me in general, and for their endless enthusiasm as pioneers in the field of cardiac rehabilitation.

Jacqueline Wehmueller, editor at the Johns Hopkins University Press, for her kindness, her guidance, her competence, her belief in this book, and her true understanding of what I have tried to convey.

Ann Walston, for her friendship, her advice about publishing, her talent in book design, and her foresight in leading me to the Johns Hopkins University Press.

Anne Herndon, Ph.D., my valued friend and colleague, for her most helpful comments and encouragement.

Al Julian, Ph.D., for his thoughtful and thorough editing of my initial manuscript.

Patty Farrell, M.D., and Frank Farrell, M.D., for their enthusiasm about this project and their painstaking review of my initial work.

Jack Rejeski, Ph.D., for his helpful review of my manuscript and hints about the publishing process.

Barry Franklin, Ph.D., and Kathy Berra, B.S.N., for their early reviews and support of this work.

Herb Soper, M.D., for his helpful information regarding female sexuality.

Deborah Lynn Farmer, for her help in manuscript preparation and for generally putting up with me.

Lynn Swaim, for her insistence that readers don't need M.D.'s or Ph.D.'s to understand well-written manuscripts, and for her ever-present Tuesday wit and smiles.

The staff at the Wake Forest Cardiac Rehabilitation Program, for making my work in cardiac rehab the most enjoyable part of my professional life.

And the nice people at the Johns Hopkins University Press for making the publishing of this book a gracious and joyful experience.

Introduction

∎ ∎ ∎ ∎ ∎ ∎

This is not a book about cholesterol or diet management. It does not discuss treadmill testing, or how to quit smoking, or any of the other aspects of cardiac rehabilitation that are typically written about. Although those aspects of health care are important and necessary in recovering from heart disease, limiting the discussion of living with heart illness to those topics overlooks a nearly universal truth: illness does not affect only individuals; illness disrupts families.

Unfortunately, relatively little attention has been paid to this topic. Neither professional nor popular literature has addressed the emotional pains and stresses faced by heart patients and their loved ones as they struggle with cardiac rehabilitation. Far too little help has been offered to cardiac couples as they have watched their marriages and family relationships fill with the fears, anger, guilt, and regrets that inevitably develop when people are living with heart illness.

For some couples and families, these pressures ruin intimacy. When people are coping with illness, marriages and families can become arenas of tension. Unexpressed and unfulfilled needs and subtle or open power struggles often lead cardiac couples into lives of quiet desperation. What a pity! At a time in life when each spouse is most in need of the kind of soothing and nurturing that can come only from a loving partner, emotional distance and loneliness accumulate instead.

Fortunately, other couples report a very different family experience in coping with heart disease. For them, the shock of illness is a needed slap in the face that gets the attention of every family member. Prior unexpressed feelings get expressed. Unforgiven hurts are soothed, and forgiveness leads to renewed emotional closeness. Positive aspects of life are emphasized and shared, unhealthy habits are changed, and intimacy grows. Such couples and their families begin living each day to the fullest. For them, coping with heart illness actually stirs changes that improve relationships.

What makes the difference? How can you help one another to fall into the second category of couples and families? How can you help each other and yourself to cope with the often overwhelming series of physical and emotional tasks called "living with heart disease" and not let the coping kill your spirit of caring in the process? These are the topics explored in this book.

As director of psychological services at the Wake Forest University Cardiac Rehabilitation Program and a clinical psychologist specializing in marriage and family therapy, I have had a unique opportunity to learn about the psychological effect of heart illness on both individuals and relationships. I have had the privilege—and sometimes the agony—of spending literally thousands of hours over the past thirteen years privy to many individual and relationship struggles to cope with heart disease. The hundreds of individuals and couples who have allowed me to share in their intimate journeys of rehabilitation have taught me much. My main lessons have involved learning to recognize the differences between the people who experience heart illness as the beginning of the end of family intimacy and those who react to it in ways that improve their personal relationships.

The pages that follow will guide you and your loved ones in your efforts to manage your own, and to understand each other's, emotional reactions to heart illness and to cardiac rehabilitation. Throughout this book I discuss strategies and concepts that I have found helpful in controlling marital and family reactions to illness. Key among the concepts are these notions: (1) families are teams that are run by the marriage partners; and (2) the entire family is affected whenever individual members are undergoing stressful changes.

I also discuss illness as a stressor that stirs individual psychological reactions that must be understood and controlled if marriages are to grow. In this discussion, I present multiple guidelines for managing the stress of illness within your personal life, whether you are a heart patient or the concerned partner of a heart patient.

I have tried to write the kind of book that will be of use to a wide variety of couples. No two marriages are exactly alike, and the psychological effects of cardiac rehabilitation vary depending on the unique factors that distinguish your marriage. Throughout this book I have incorporated numerous case examples of various types of heart illness and types of families. I know I have not captured every conceivable variation in these examples; to do so would be impossible. But I do hope you will find the descriptions of these problems helpful in further understanding your unique family situation. I hope you will find comfort in knowing that other people have gone through experiences similar to yours. But beyond this, I sincerely hope you will benefit from the practical advice that I offer.

Finally, I would like to say that I have written this book to apply to all cardiac couples, regardless of whether husband or wife is the heart patient. Other works have addressed the specific struggles faced by women in coping with their husbands' heart conditions. I believe certain differences do exist between the struggles typically faced by wives and by husbands coping with a mate's heart illness. However, most of the marital struggles faced by cardiac couples are universal, regardless of which member of the couple is the heart patient.

To my knowledge, this is the first published work that has addressed cardiac rehabilitation from a truly marital perspective. I hope that reading this book will be the start of new and better chapters in your rehabilitation and in your marriage.

Part I

· · · · · ·

The Family as a Team in Sickness and in Health

One

A Family in Distress

∎ ∎ ∎ ∎ ∎ ∎

Maria Hinson* was referred to me by her family doctor for stress management training. Maria, who was fifty-three years old, had been suffering from incapacitating migraine headaches for nine months prior to referral. She had recently begun having trouble sleeping and had lost fourteen pounds even though she was not dieting. It was obvious that Maria was depressed. In our initial interview, Maria shared with me her confusion about her physician's suggestion that her problems might be stress related. She described herself as happily married to a loving husband and as a person who generally enjoyed life. She and her spouse were proud of their successful family business, which was now being run by their only child, twenty-four-year-old John.

Maria did admit that she had undergone "quite a scare" three years earlier, when her husband had suffered a "moderately serious" heart attack. She emphasized, however, that her spouse's physical recovery had been uncomplicated and that he had breezed through subsequent triple coronary artery bypass surgery. Maria did not see that her husband's illness and recovery had any relationship to her current difficulties. She emphasized that she and her family had made "various

---

*Throughout this book I cite case examples drawn from my clinical experiences. Out of respect for my patients' privacy, I have changed the names and identifying characteristics of every person described in this book.

necessary adjustments" in reacting to the illness. In her opinion, all was running smoothly in her life now, so why all this talk about stress?

As our interview continued, I focused on the "various necessary adjustments" that Maria and her family had implemented in reacting to her husband's illness. She explained that her spouse, Henry, had had a history of struggling with depression before his heart attack. She stated that Henry was a true mystery. On the one hand, he was an ambitious, energetic, self-made man who prided himself on meeting life's challenges head-on. But Henry was also a chronic worrier who stressed himself into periods of agitated depression by quietly obsessing about all that might go wrong in life. When he had his heart attack, Maria and John became understandably afraid that Henry would "worry himself into another depression and never recover." In reaction to their fear of Henry's potential for relapsing, Maria and John adopted what seemed to be a good strategy of preventive medicine: in hopes of keeping Henry from worrying himself into depression, they decided to buffer him from all stress.

John, who was a junior in college at the time of Henry's heart attack, promptly withdrew from school and returned home to run the family business. Maria devoted herself to running interference for Henry around the house. When bills came, she intercepted them and paid them without telling Henry; when the furnace burned out, she bought a new one and arranged for it to be installed "without bothering Henry with the aggravation of the details." She particularly made sure not to "worry and scare" Henry with any discussion of her headaches, insomnia, or weight loss.

I asked Maria how this antidepressant strategy that she and her son had cooked up was working. With fatigue in her voice and tears in her eyes she quietly discussed her continued love and growing concern for her husband. Henry seemed to be miserable. He had aged noticeably since his heart attack and surgery. He seemed to be disinterested in life; not exactly depressed, but generally melancholy and unresponsive. He seldom laughed, and he was acting more withdrawn and preoccupied with each passing month.

Maria cried as she described how much she missed her husband's shining wit and energizing zest for meeting the challenges of each new day. She blushed and apologized as though she had spoken forbidden words when she admitted her longing for more romantic and sexual playfulness of the sort that she and Henry had always enjoyed before his heart illness. As she put it, "Even during his periods of depression, Henry and I could always block out the world and escape into the privacy of our love and passion for each other. Those times always kept us going; now, they are gone."

Maria's primary source of emotional support since Henry's illness had been her son. She and John jointly made decisions regarding the family business, and they spent many hours discussing their shared concerns about Henry. Mother and son had recently decided that it might be good for Henry if he and Maria began to travel. They hoped that Henry's mood would brighten if he reconnected with old friends and relatives from whom he had grown distant during the busy years of establishing and running his business.

As our interview continued, I expressed concern and admiration for Maria's son; he seemed quite young for the responsibilities he had shouldered during the past several years. This time Maria's tears and words were those of a concerned and frightened parent who did not quite want to believe the refrain that echoed throughout her private moments of motherly reflection.

When John quit college, he had been engaged to be married, but his relationship with his fiancée, who had remained in school, withered and ended within a year. John showed no sadness; he just worked harder to learn the family business. He did have many friends from his high-school days, and he socialized to a reasonable degree. However, he did not date much, and he generally filled his life trying to take up the slack created by his father's illness. Maria was particularly concerned for John of late because he had been suffering from "chronic indigestion." He had recently undergone various medical tests to investigate what his doctors were calling a preulcerative condition.

Maria summarized her concerns for her son: "I know he's just a kid who's been forced to live a man's life. But I don't know what we can do to make this better right now." Our first session ended with Maria's agreeing to my meeting with her husband next.

Henry was a well-dressed man with a powerful presence, but he looked rather tired and uncomfortably unsure of himself. The way he combined a powerful personal presence with awkwardness and vulnerability reminded me of how a great football coach looks on television when he is being interviewed after his team has lost a major game. It soon became apparent that Henry's discomfort was largely due to his suspicion that Maria had arranged this meeting with me as an indirect way of getting him to come for psychological counseling. He stated that Maria's taking control of his life "for his own sake" would have been par for the course, given the way their marriage had been since his heart attack. Henry very clearly did not like the spectator role that he had been assigned and had assumed in his family and his business during the past three years. In his words:

"Yes, I had a heart attack and bypass surgery three years ago, but my wife and son act as if I'd *died* three years ago. Bills come to my house and my wife hides them from me, like I'm going to believe that we now live debt free if I don't see the checkbook. My son, who didn't know a profit-and-loss statement from a lost-and-found station, all of a sudden quit college without consulting me and moved into *my* office at the building that *I* built to house the business that *I* created.

"Now, don't misunderstand; I love and appreciate Maria and John. I know they're doing what they think is best for me, and I guess they're following my doctor's orders. But they must know something about my condition that I don't know. I simply do not feel ready to be put out to pasture. Hell, I'm only fifty-nine years old!"

What is wrong with this picture? This very nice family is floundering waist deep in a swamp of emotional pain. At this time, when they most need and want their family relations to be sources of healing to one another, they are actually drowning in their mounting tensions, frustrations, and fears.

The Hinsons are caught in a family trap. Their attempted solutions to feared problems are actually making things worse. The hierarchy of authority that once organized this family is now in a shambles. The marriage that should be the core of this family team is dwindling in intimacy. The stresses felt by each of these good people are accumulating and ruining everyone's health. Their growth and development as individuals and as a family and a couple have been frozen by the stresses caused by the flurry of changes that began with Henry's heart attack. Communication is diminishing and despair is mounting for the Hinsons.

What could these people have done differently? More important, what can they now do to repair and reorganize their marital and family relationships? The following pages present information that can be used to answer these questions. By understanding the unique and fascinating ways marriages and families work—in sickness and in health—perhaps you can avoid the pitfalls that have trapped good families like the Hinsons.

Two

The Many Stresses of Illness

■ ■ ■ ■ ■ ■

*T*he necessary beginning point in understanding your own and your loved ones' psychological reactions to heart illness is to understand that illness is a *stressor*—a stimulus that causes stress. *Stress* is what happens psychologically and physically whenever you are faced with the need to adapt or to adjust behaviorally, emotionally, or physically.

Heart illness is a stressor that does not discriminate; it strikes with no regard for your frame of mind, life situation, or degree of readiness. Once it strikes, heart illness changes your life and your marriage forever. For the heart patient, the immediate change from being "well" to being "recovering" cuts to the core of self-concept and self-esteem. Just as rapidly, the patient's loved ones are shocked into a flood of emotions and a flurry of activities in reaction to the illness.

Consider for a moment the phenomenal number of adjustments faced by any individual or family suddenly confronted with this illness. Changes brought about by heart illness include, but are not limited to

- strange physical symptoms that leave you feeling out of control of your own body;

- a flood of preoccupation with death and, sometimes, overwhelming fears of death;
- immediate awareness of a new set of worries about your future ability to resume normal activities and to adjust to any lingering physical effects of this illness;
- sudden disruption of customary daily life-style, including participation in work, friendship, and family circles;
- obsessive questioning about why this illness occurred, what might have been done to prevent it from happening, or what needs to be done now to prevent a recurrence;
- dependence on the unfamiliar and often confusing environments of hospitals and doctors' offices and the people who work there (the medical staff);
- consumption of medications that often make you feel and act strangely.

All this, and I have not even mentioned the endless volley of stressors that are faced upon leaving the hospital and attempting to resume a normal day-to-day life.

Remember that all these stressors affect every family member in one way or another. The heart patient, of course, is the prime target of concern and is certainly the most vulnerable at first. But the patient is also the family member who receives the most targeted reassurance, consistent medical attention, and pharmacologic help in dealing with the fear and anxiety that occur throughout this time.

Although this intense focus on the patient is certainly necessary, merited, and deserved, it is important to remember that the family members of this patient—especially the spouse—are also faced with the stressors outlined above. Unfortunately, family members are not typically identified as "patients" in this process; they are viewed neither by themselves nor by others as needing the special care and attention that come with being sick. These concerned and involved loved ones are left to manage overwhelming stress without the aid of structured monitoring, charted progress, and nurturing permission and insistence from others to "Take good care of yourself."

So here is my first major point: *Coping with heart illness involves both spouses dealing with an endless series of stressors.* Rehabilitation is not an event with a clear beginning, middle, and ending; rehabilitation is a process that begins with the onset of illness and lasts for the rest of your life. The obvious question, therefore, is not whether you and your family will be affected by this process but *how* you will manage this unique and overwhelming series of changes in your lives, especially in your marriage.

As you read on, remember that (1) no couple adjusts to heart illness with total emotional smoothness and (2) not every couple has dramatic negative reactions to heart illness. Some couples change only gradually in reaction to the stresses that result from illness. Instead of falling into open conflict and chaos, some couples simply begin to bicker more or to show more impatience in dealing with each other.

Given the numbers of stressors faced in this process, it's a wonder that any marriage survives cardiac rehabilitation. Periods of intense anxiety and depression are par for the course during the first several months of adjusting to heart illness. However, many individuals, like the Hinson family from chapter 1, get stuck in this painful first stage of adjustment. Marriage and family life then begin to revolve around intimacy-draining emotions.

In contrast, many people just seem to float through this same period and these same scary transitions with amazing ease and calmness. Some families seem to be made up of individuals who finesse their way past the multiple hurdles thrown in their path by heart illness and who run the course of recovery without accumulating emotional bumps and bruises. Many couples actually report improvement in their relationship as a result of the many changes brought on by cardiac rehabilitation.

What determines these very different reactions to what is essentially the same stressor? The simple truth is that marriages that are intimate and healthy are better able to survive stressful times. It is also true that heart patients who live in intimate marriages are better able to manage the stresses of recovery.

I do not mean to imply that you can manage the stress of recovery *for* each other. No matter how much you love and nurture each other, you each must ultimately assume responsibility for your own emotional adjustment and for changing your life-style in ways that will improve your health. No matter how much you care, you cannot eat right, stop smoking, exercise, manage stress, or keep a positive attitude toward life *for* someone else. On the other hand, it is important to remember that you have only two basic choices in being married: you will be either a source of healing or a source of stress to your partner. How you treat each other has much to do with your reactions to the stresses of life, including the stresses of living with heart illness.

In the following pages, I describe how marriages and families work and what can be done to control the particularly stressful impacts of heart illness. Use the following chapters to stimulate your thinking about your own dealings with the many aspects of cardiac rehabilitation. Also note the concerns about your partner that come to mind as you read. Throughout your reading, discuss your reactions and your concerns with each other.

If you are having difficulties in your marriage, let the information in this book challenge you to become more cooperative teammates in developing a healing partnership. If you are among the many lucky couples who are working positively together in recovering from illness, use this book as a framework for better understanding what you are doing that is working so well.

Three

Family Teams

■ ■ ■ ■ ■ ■

*M*ost of us do not live our lives solo; we live in close-knit teams called families. The cocaptains of the family team are the parents. What affects one part of the team has an overall effect on the whole team, and the rules and operations of the team—especially the rules and operations of the parents' marriage—have a great effect on each individual team member.

Family reactions and a patient's responses to cardiac rehabilitation are intimately related. There is no neutral position regarding the family's impact on the recovering heart patient; family reactions either help or hinder the patient's recovery. Just as important, but too often overlooked, is the fact that no heart patient's recovery process fails to change the family in which this recovery is taking place.

Because we are taught neither how to cope with the stresses of illness nor how to work together as family teammates, it is a rare family that does not make mistakes in reacting to illness. The effects of these mistakes can complicate the heart patient's recovery and can lead to some part of the family team breaking down.

If you and your family are stuck in unhealthy reactions to illness, the accumulated tensions are probably causing symptoms someplace in your family. These symptoms might appear either in individual family members or in relationships between certain family members. In the case example of the Hinsons, both types of symptoms were evident: Maria and her son were showing physical signs of stress, and Maria's relationship with her husband was obviously losing sexual and emotional intimacy.

Of tremendous concern to me are those families who do not show any obvious signs of stress in reacting to illness but who settle into a subtle and dangerous shift in their ways of living as a family. These people appear to be doing a lot better than they actually are. At first, there may be no open conflict in the family or blatant symptoms shown by any individual member. Or the family may simply be failing to notice the signals of distress that are being sent out and that are obvious to observers outside the family. In either case, such families often settle into ways of interacting that undermine coping ability and health. For these families, illness behavior often becomes the focus of family life.

I once worked with the wife of a heart patient whose comments succinctly described this family dilemma. Without realizing it, she and her family had begun living a life that focused on illness rather than on wellness. She described herself and her family this way:

"After my husband's heart attack, we all got used to walking on eggshells in dealing with him. He was afraid he wouldn't recover, and we didn't really know exactly what to do to help him. We all changed our lives in umpteen ways out of fear of his 'weak heart.' We basically stopped doing anything but work, worry, and wait for the next heart attack.

"The strange thing is that none of us realized how much we had changed. Life got pretty miserable for us all, but we just kept on plowing through and never talked about how unhappy we all were. Our daughter's divorce shocked us all into looking at how we had been living our lives. We realized that this man was likely to survive his heart attack but kill us all in the process!"

To control the impact of illness on your family, it is important to understand how families operate as teams.

How Families Work

Just like individuals, families are creatures of habit; they resist change. We grow accustomed to enacting the roles that we have been assigned and that we have assumed in our families, and these ways of relating come to feel natural. For example, Little Brother always remains Little Brother in family gatherings, even if he does happen to be fifty-nine years old, twice as intelligent, and three times as wealthy as the rest of the family. Consequently, adjusting to new circumstances (such as illness) is very difficult for families. The Johnsons are a case in point.

Claudia Johnson was a patient at the Wake Forest University Cardiac Rehabilitation Program who set records for her extremely high cholesterol levels. She was friendly and cooperative in general, but her refusal to follow through with our recommendations about her obvious need to change her diet was confusing to us all. Then we interviewed her husband.

Ed Johnson explained that his wife was the youngest of four daughters from a very close family. Her "family role" had always been that of the good-natured fat sister who loved to eat. Claudia's family was filled with people who believed that the key to good health was to eat food that sticks to your ribs. Accordingly, her family tradition was filled with meals loaded with eggs, red meat, and starches. In addition, the patriarch of Claudia's family—her paternal grandfather—was legendary within the family for having lived to be ninety-one years old although he "ate four eggs and smoked a pack of unfiltered cigarettes every day."

As a natural show of their loving concern, Claudia's family kept her well supplied with country hams, baked desserts, and other traditional family favorites. Ed tried to explain tactfully to his wife's family that what Claudia really needed from them was support and encouragement to change her diet, not encouragement to eat herself to death. The family responded with a clear message that he did not know what was best for Claudia. They reminded him that their family and all its traditions had been a part of Claudia's life far longer than Ed had.

Throughout the first year of Claudia's recovery, Ed seethed in fear and anger at his wife for not being more assertive about refusing her family's food. He accused her of caring more about what her siblings, aunts, and uncles thought of her than about her own health or her own marriage. He finally stopped arguing with her and became re-signed to the fact that he could not change her. He explained, "It's just too much to ask her to go against her family tradition and not show appreciation to these people by refusing their food; that's just not who she is. I don't like it, but I can't change it."

Although the potential medical complications of following such family rules are obvious, the way to deal with the emotional discom-fort that comes from trying to change age-old family patterns is not so obvious. But by learning about two important factors that influence the workings of your family, you can better control your family reac-tions. These factors are *the circular family dance* and *family structure*.

The Circular Family Dance

Have you ever asked yourself why we experience the same old prob-lems in relating to each other, year after year? Or why in the world we do not come to some new answers to these problems that keep pla-guing us? Why *do* couples keep having the same old nonproductive fights about sex, money, in-laws, children, or whatever?

Unfortunately, we tend to get stuck in vicious circles of interaction in close relationships. The more we try to solve a problem by using a certain strategy, the worse the problem gets. The worse the problem gets, the harder we try the same old strategy. When this happens, our attempts to solve anticipated problems in relationships often do noth-ing but fuel the feared problem.

The Hinson family from chapter 1 beautifully demonstrates this point. Out of fear that Henry would be depressed, Maria and their son, John, began to run interference for Henry. As a result, Henry began to feel left out of the family, and he became depressed. The more de-pressed Henry acted, the more Maria and John ran interference. The more interference, the more depression; and so on.

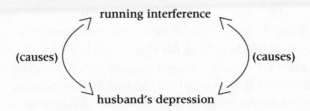

The higher your stress level, the more likely you are to get stuck in a self-perpetuating mess rather than try a new strategy. When you are faced with stress, you automatically reach for ways of coping that feel natural. You tend to use your familiar coping strategies harder and harder, regardless of whether the strategies are working to help you get what you want.

An obviously healthier choice would be to pay attention to the outcome that is resulting from your attempts to influence each other. If you are not getting the reactions you want, try this revolutionary idea: *Do something different!*

Once Henry and Maria began talking directly to each other about their shared concerns over what was happening in their marriage and family, Henry's depression lifted. Maria correspondingly began to back off from running interference. Her stress levels lessened, and the burdens placed on her son as the family savior lightened as Henry became reinvolved in his life. The key to this positive change in the Hinson family was their willingness to confront their circular patterns and to try something different.

Family Structure

An often subtle form of circular dance that happens in some families involves confusing the family structure. Families run according to rules. Some of these rules are obviously stated and serve as clear guidelines for interacting with one another. Other rules are felt or assumed but not spoken out loud. Whether obvious or subtle, these rules determine how family members interact; these rules structure the family.

Healthy families have clear and sensible rules that structure the relationships within the family. Key among these rules is that the parents share more and greater varieties of intimacy with each other than either shares with any other family member. The "mother of family therapy," the late Virginia Satir, once commented, "The marital relationship is the axis around which all other family relationships are formed. The mates are the 'architects' of the family."[1] This rule should continue to apply regardless of the ages of your children. It is certainly true and appropriate that as parents age, they may become more dependent on their grown children. However, healthy families continue to respect the rule that parents have a right to privacy and the now grown children have a right to live their own lives.

Periodically I have the delightful experience of addressing the residents of a local retirement home about the marital and family issues that are encountered during the years of senior adulthood. One of these residents bragged to me about the closeness that had developed between him and his four grown children in recent years, especially since the death of their mother five years before. When asked to share the secret of this success, he replied: "One thing my children don't do is forget about me for long periods of time. One thing I don't do is forget that my children have their own families now and that they sometimes need my encouragement to forget about me for a while."

The point to underscore is that *stress tends to disrupt family structure;* it changes the ways family members relate to one another. These changes in relationship patterns can lead to a variety of problems.

One unhealthy pattern that is typical in families coping with illness involves two members becoming emotionally close at the expense of a third member. This pattern can be a particular problem if the two closely connected family members are from different generations in the family hierarchy; for example, a parent and a child may get close but exclude the other parent. When this happens, it almost always leads to such tension within the family that someone or some relationship is damaged. Once again, I refer to the Hinson family as an example.

Maria and Henry suffered a breakdown of marital intimacy, and

---

[1]V. Satir, *Conjoint Family Therapy* (Palo Alto, Calif.: Science and Behavior Books, 1964), p. 1.

everyone involved developed symptoms of stress as Maria turned primarily to her son, rather than to her husband, for emotional support. Although the excessive joining between the child and one parent in this family was well-intentioned, it confused the overall teamwork and comfort that is necessary for healthy family functioning. The Hinsons broke an important family rule, and they paid a high price. Fortunately, they changed in time to avoid bankrupting their family's emotional fortunes.

Following my session with Henry Hinson, I met with him and his wife together. I encouraged them to begin discussing with each other the same concerns that they each had shared openly with me. Fortunately, they were willing to try this different way of relating to the fears and concerns that had paralyzed their marriage since Henry's heart attack.

But they did not just talk; they found the courage to change. First, they made a list of the many responsibilities and concerns that faced them as a couple: business matters, household financial responsibilities, management of retirement funds, dealings with insurance companies and with Henry's doctors, needed areas of change in their family diet and other life-style matters, the day-to-day running of the household, and, of course, their son, John.

John accompanied them to their next counseling session and was lovingly included in planning how this family would go about changing. The therapy setting was helpful in pointing out to the Hinsons the many ways in which they had created an uncomfortable family structure, one in which Mom and Son were running Dad's life. The relief and the appreciation that this family felt toward one another as they openly discussed their life together was obvious and touching.

For several weeks, Maria and Henry grappled with various possible ways of restructuring their life. They included their son in some of these discussions, but they often expressed their thoughts, feelings, and wishes privately, as husband and wife—just like old times. The Hinsons decided that Henry would indeed remain retired from running his business. Instead of working outside the home, he would take over managing the household and family finances, his own paperwork with his medical insurance companies, and the day-to-day operations of the household. He expressed a new enthusiasm for learning to cook—a part of family life that Maria had never really enjoyed, anyway.

Free of the pressures of running their home, Maria found that she could better manage the pressures of running their family business, but she admitted that she needed help in this area. This time, both Henry and Maria were clear that this help needed to come from someone other than their son. They decided to hire a business manager.

Maria and Henry emphasized to their son their sincere hope that he would return to college and finish his education. John reacted honestly: he did not feel ready or motivated to return to school, but neither did he particularly enjoy working in the family business. Instead, he opted to get a job in a company that employed several of his high-school friends. He also stated that he wanted to begin sharing an apartment with these buddies.

I do not mean to imply that the Hinsons changed easily or that they just went on to live happily ever after. Like all families, they continued to have times of struggle and disappointment. Seven years after his first operation, Henry had to undergo bypass surgery again. Maria still periodically suffers stress-related headaches, and she feels sadness and resentment because her life plan has been changed by Henry's heart illness. John never did return to complete his education, and his efforts to establish a career outside his family business have not succeeded. But these family crises and disappointments were met head-on by this couple. They are no longer stuck in attempted solutions that do not work, and they no longer mess up their family structure in facing their stressful times.

There is another troublesome family structure, one that is found in some families that operate quite differently from the way the Hinsons do. Here, family members grow accustomed to keeping excessive emotional distance from one another. They simply do not nurture or soothe one another; nor do they communicate or cooperate among themselves. Everyone lives in emotional disconnection. Such families have much difficulty feeling comfortable in reacting to crises such as illness. The obvious need for healing through intimate connections during such times makes these families uncomfortable. They tend either to flounder in awkwardness as they attempt to be more caring, or to seethe in guilt and anger over not giving or receiving more nurturance.

Summary

Family teams resist change.

Families tend to dance circular dances.

Family structures are important in determining how we relate to one another.

Bearing these factors in mind, we turn now to a closer examination of healthy and unhealthy family reactions to illness.

Four

Healthy Family
Reactions to Illness

∙ ∙ ∙ ∙ ∙ ∙

*W*ith whom do you compare yourselves when you are deciding how well you are adjusting to illness? Notice that my question implies that such a comparison is inevitable. Consciously or not, we tend to evaluate ourselves by observing how others appear to be. Based on such comparisons, some people settle for what is actually a poor way of coping. As the case example of the Johnsons demonstrated, the family tradition may dictate that you act a certain way, but that is not necessarily the wise way to act. Continuing in these family ways might feel right because such ways of relating to one another and to the world are familiar. But this feeling of familiarity does not necessarily mean you are making wise choices in your current life.

Perhaps even more typical is the tendency to compare your marriage and family negatively with some imagined standard of perfection; feeling bad is the inevitable consequence. Somehow, other families just seem to struggle less, enjoy more, and manage better than the people who are living under your own roof.

Much of my counseling with cardiac couples involves teaching them to use realistic standards in their self-analysis. Without accurate information about what is healthy, you run the risk of making one or both of the preceding mistakes; you might discount your own goodness, or you might accept as normal a form of family functioning that is actually impaired.

I have included the following descriptions of healthy family reactions to illness to give you a realistic picture with which you can compare yourselves. However, as you read on, you must remember one thing: *There are no perfect families.*

Even the healthiest families may react to the shock of illness with periods of distress, disorganization, and conflict. Therefore, the initial stages of family adjustments to illness are often similar in families with healthy coping patterns and in families with unhealthy coping patterns. What distinguishes these two groups is how the family ultimately responds to the disruption caused by illness.

Healthy families can be described as progressing through three stages of reaction while adjusting to the illness of a loved one. Each stage has certain behavioral, emotional, and interpersonal characteristics.

Initial Stage: Let's Get Together and Endure

When a loved one first gets sick, most families band together and simply try to get through day by day. At first, family members buffer their shock by becoming numb and by focusing on one another in caring and concerned ways as they await the outcome of the crisis. The question of whether the loved one will survive haunts everyone until this initial stage passes.

The emotional wounds that must eventually be healed during recovery from heart illness begin with the hospitalizing of the heart patient. It is as traumatic to see a loved one go through this frightening experience as it is to go through it yourself. The siren screams as the ambulance speeds off, and your life is changed forever. Soon you are confronted with the bustling and disorienting environment of the hospital. Monitors beep, heart rates are graphed as squiggly lines on television screens, and tubes seem to be attached everywhere. The patient and the family are separated as the medical team takes charge of a life that is precious to you all. Time seems endless as the drama with an unclear outcome—life or death?—unfolds.

If surgery is required, there is the additional horror of life on a respirator. The patient cannot speak and may float in and out of aware-ness. The patient's frustrations and fears at being unable to communi-cate with nurses and loved ones are frightening. For the family, the image of a loved one lying helpless—connected to a machine, with tubes coming out of nose and throat, and needles dripping fluids into both arms—can last a lifetime. Such memories haunt Warren from the time his wife had bypass surgery: "Rebecca was always so full of life and energy. I had never seen her sick. When I saw her for the first time after her bypass operation, I truly thought *I* would have a heart attack. I was afraid to touch her. She didn't look like my wife. I still feel guilty about this, but the truth is that I was glad she was asleep. I had to leave the room after just a few minutes."

Fortunately, 98 percent of patients who have bypass surgery sur-vive. But the family drama does not end with transfer from the critical care unit to the general cardiac floor. Once the patient is reasonably stable, the family is faced with the helplessness of being unable to cure their loved one. Feelings of relief are mixed with panic, fear, and sad-ness that this illness has happened.

Most people soon begin to be plagued with feelings of guilt. The guilt takes various forms:

"I should have kept this from happening."

"I wish we had settled our differences before this happened."

"I can't believe I let this happen to myself; now I'll be a big bother to everyone."

"I feel terrible about the argument we had yesterday" (or last week, or last year, or five years ago).

"I can't remember the last time I said 'I love you' out loud."

Healthy families are able to express such feelings openly, and they respond nurturingly to each other. But family tensions inevitably mount during this phase, both because of the stress of the situation and because the heart patient may remain somewhat withdrawn and unresponsive to others. This withdrawal is often an effect of medica-tion; it may also be the psychological defense of blocking out the over-whelming emotional impact of a serious medical crisis. Unfortunately, the patient's withdrawal collides with the emotional needs of the frightened family. Family members want proof that the patient is going to recover and that their efforts to soothe and help the patient are working; at the same time, however, the patient may be less than willing or able to discuss these matters with *anyone*.

Thus, family members often develop feelings of anger and frustration. These feelings are fueled by the fatigue that soon sets in from keeping hospital vigils. The stressed and tired family may take their frustrations out on one another, noting who is reacting more or less caringly to everyone else during the ordeal.

More often, the tensions are taken out on medical personnel. The doctors and nurses just never seem to do or care enough to be helpful to the sick family member. The doctors and nurses may indeed be uncaring and unavailable, but it is also likely that no amount of care could cure the real pain that flows through families at this time: heartache and a desperate wish that this had not happened.

Intermediate Stage: Developing a Game Plan

Once the shock of the initial diagnosis or hospitalization has passed, families become more task oriented in their coping efforts. Now family members begin aggressively to seek specific information about the patient's condition and the anticipated course of treatment, hospitalization, and rehabilitation. Many of these important questions have no definite medical answers, and this uncertainty increases frustration and fear among family members. This is the stage during which difficult emotions surface in families. Reactions to the tensions of the situation can begin hurting marriages during this stage, too. One of the most difficult aspects of this stage is dealing with grief.

Major illness is always equated with loss, and grieving begins immediately. This is not to imply that every cardiac family experiences the wailing-and-gnashing-of-teeth variety of mourning. Many heart patients and their families report a kind of grieving that is more like melancholia, in which they become preoccupied with thoughts about the meaning of their lives—past, present, and future.

For others, illness brings a grieving process that is similar to what happens when a loved one actually dies. *Denial* and *shock* over this illness, and the feared losses of health and of a happy and healthy future, lead to periods of *despair* and *confusion*. Next comes a period of *bargaining*—the grieving individual clings to the fantasy that the loss can be erased "if I can just be good enough" in following the rules of rehabilitation. Of course, the bargaining stage inevitably ends in disappointment. Neither the illness nor the need for rehabilitation goes away. Stages of *anger* and *sadness* then follow. These painful emotions must be identified and fully expressed before the grief can progress to *acceptance*.

In healthy families, grieving is done out loud. Family members express their feelings within earshot of one another. It is a mistake to hold back expression of feelings of grief and sadness during stressful times. Doing so only increases your pain and distances you from your family. Allowing a loved one the privilege of seeing and hearing your most private reactions is an act that demonstrates your love, respect, and trust for that person. The fears, worries, and tender feelings experienced during this stage of adjustment need to be shared within families.

A myth that works against emotional healing in dealing with heart illness is the notion that the patient might die from experiencing any strong emotion or from seeing his or her spouse show any strong feelings. Although it is wise to avoid emotional excitement during the immediate stage of recovering from illness, you should know that few heart patients die from excitement. In fact, in families that believe this myth, the heart patient might feel "dead" from the boredom of being shut out of intimate interchanges with loved ones!

The truth is that holding in emotions is much more stressful for any individual patient, and growing distant from your mate because of failure to be open is much more stressful for couples. Holding back expression of feelings in your marriage will only contribute to a growing sense of depression for each of you. Healthy couples are open with each other about their feelings—even their grief, anger, and frustrations about illness.

At this stage, couples often begin grappling with tensions that have to do with their reactions to medical treatment. By now, the patient is out of shock and is no longer sedated, probably growing frustrated and expressing aggravations over inadequate medical care to the spouse more often than to anyone else. The problem is that the spouse feels powerless to make this problem go away and may feel placed in an uncomfortable double bind: afraid that complaining to the medical personnel might alienate them; afraid that *not* complaining might alienate the sick spouse.

Tensions often grow in the marriage as the spouse and other family members continue to shield the patient from accurate and honest information about his or her condition. This pattern may be indirectly encouraged by the behavior of medical personnel. When a doctor or nurse takes the spouse and family aside and quietly discusses the patient's condition, the indirect message being given is, "It would be better for the patient not to hear these facts." Although shielding the patient from the truth is well-intentioned, it soon proves to be far more frustrating, frightening, and insulting to the patient than it is helpful.

The first round of what often becomes an ongoing source of marital tension in cardiac rehabilitation begins now—differences in interpretations of medical advice. That a husband and wife might interpret doctors' advice differently is certainly understandable when you consider how some of the medical advice is given. What, after all, is specifically meant by such phrases as "Use in moderation" or "Begin to exercise at your own pace" or "Use your own judgment"? Furthermore, the initial instructions for at-home rehabilitation procedures and facts about the patient's condition are given during the stress-filled period of hospitalization. This is, understandably, a time when spouse and patient are not at their best in terms of digesting new information.

We often see patients in our outpatient cardiac rehabilitation program who swear that they were given no input about diet, exercise, sex, work, and other matters upon being discharged from the hospital. The truth most often is that the information was offered but did not register in the minds of the couple, both of whom were still reeling in semishock. When husband and wife don't agree about what is and is not safe or advisable behavior, conflict between the couple is fueled. What often happens next is that the spouse begins to monitor the patient's behavior like a parent looking over the shoulder of a child. This, of course, quickly becomes tiresome for both partners and leads to direct or indirect bickering.

Such marital tensions often lead to both the heart patient and the spouse experiencing a period of depression shortly after returning home from the hospital. This homecoming depression usually lifts within four to six weeks, more or less. Healthy couples help each other through this phase by allowing each other freedom to vent feelings and by giving each other ample support and reassurance that life will go on.

Long-Range Adjustment: Coping Together

All does not remain tense and chaotic for healthy couples, regardless of the stresses being faced. After returning home and getting through the initial months of recovery from the hospital experience, healthy couples actually restore intimacy within their relationship, and order in their family operations, rather quickly. Of course, they continue to struggle with the stresses of rehabilitation, but they begin to do so with a renewed sense of teamwork. How quickly the family heals is directly related to two factors: (1) the stress level of the couple at the time the illness strikes and (2) the amount of change the illness generates within the family.

This makes common sense; a family that is already fatigued by stresses such as financial or relationship problems will have more difficulty adjusting to the struggles of coping with illness. And any family that is turned upside down by the additional stresses that sometimes come in the wake of illness—such as increased financial pressures or having to relocate to be closer to helpful family members—will have additional hurdles to scale in the rehabilitation process. For such families, reaching a state of relative calm will take longer.

Regardless of how long it takes to develop healthy adjustment, certain marital and family factors signal that healthy adjustment has been achieved:

- Flexibly adjusting family roles and rules.
- Allowing each other to react honestly.
- Seeking accurate information about rehabilitation.
- Setting clear and realistic goals.
- Coming to peace with oneself and others.

Adjusting Family Roles and Rules

Healthy couples teach their families to understand the need to be flexible in reaction to this ever-changing life. Flexibility is stronger than rigidity. In dealing with change, healthy families are able to adjust their roles and the rules that determine their reactions to one another. Healthy families are willing to change to become part of the solution to the problem they face rather than stay stuck in patterns that complicate the problem. This willingness to be flexible in adjusting roles and rules is necessary in both marital and family relations.

For example, even though the husband may always have functioned as the primary breadwinner in the family, the couple may have to adjust to the wife's working outside the home and the husband's assuming some of the domestic responsibilities now that he is medically disabled. Or even though the grandmother has always been available as a full-time baby-sitter and cook for her grandchildren, she and her family may need to adjust to the fact that she now has to devote more of her time and energy to her cardiac rehabilitation program.

Two characteristics stand out as healthy families adjust roles in reaction to illness: (1) No single family member loses because of these changes. (2) Changes are made in a way that allows the patient to keep a positive sense of self-esteem and value within the family. There are no martyrs in healthy families. To the extent possible, family problem-solving revolves around creating win-win outcomes. When a family is adjusting healthily to heart illness, no one person gets stuck with an unfair amount of the considerable stress caused by rehabilitation. Everyone continues to live a full life, even though changes in areas of responsibility may be necessary.

This point is particularly important for cardiac couples. Fears of the consequences of heart illness to loved ones often lead to two problem patterns in the family. First, the heart patient may feel guilty for putting the family through this ordeal and then overwork in an effort not to do further damage to loved ones. Feeling guilty, the patient may withdraw from activities or relationships that always used to be enjoyable and focus exclusively on work and on the task of getting well. The problem with this pattern is that lack of pleasure in life leads to irritability and depression—emotions that complicate rehabilitation.

Second, and perhaps even more typical, the patient's spouse may feel overburdened with responsibilities to be all things to all people. It is easy to drift into exhaustion from attempting to be the family's emotional cheerleader, the family dietitian, the medical liaison between patient and doctors, the head of the household, the primary wage earner, and the patient's conscience about health care habits, all at the same time.

Living under such overwhelming stress would cause anyone pain and unhappiness. Loneliness, tensions, and physical and emotional symptoms of distress are likely to result.

In coping with heart illness, it is important to be reasonably available, to be reasonably helpful to and supportive of each other. You should not feel alone in dealing with the fears of this journey, but neither should you demand excessive "rescuing" from your mate. Be flexible enough to help each other adjust to the changing roles in your marriage. Be honest with yourselves and with each other about what you need from each other. Be supportive of your mate's needs to have life involvements in areas other than cardiac rehabilitation. This is essential if your marriage is to remain healthy.

Perhaps the hallmark of the healthy couple's adjustment to illness is the ability to make changes that are realistically necessary because of the illness, but *not* to change so much that the patient ends up feeling left out of the family. Do not make the mistake the Hinsons made: the heart patient got put into the role of spectator in his own family, and he understandably became depressed when his wife and son lived stress-filled lives that excluded him.

It is important to see the heart patient's physical problems as being something of a handicap, but not as erasing the patient's worth in the operations of the family. I emphasize the importance of the family continuing to value and insist on the heart patient's participation in family operations.

It is not enough simply to convey continued love for the person who has survived the heart attack or the heart surgery—as was the case with the Hinsons. It certainly is important for family members to value one another simply for existing, but it is also important to remember that each of us requires the self-esteem that comes from being needed in tangible ways. In this vein, healthy families support and encourage the patient to participate in work and daily routine as fully as possible. A useful guideline for families that is worth repeating and remembering is this: Do for the sick family member what that person cannot do for himself or herself, and no more. By following this guideline, family members prevent heart disease from disqualifying anyone from being a valuable contributor in the overall teamwork of the family.

Each of the preceding types of changes in roles and rules leads to obvious modifications in family life. Not so obvious is yet another important variation of this theme: in coping with illness, healthy families often allow for change in the rules that dictate what kinds of thoughts and feelings get openly expressed in family interactions. That is, faced with the awareness that this is our only life—and that it is far too short—healthy family members respond to illness with increased openness and honesty in their dealings with one another. This often leads to new behavior that everyone may find both awkward and appropriate at the same time:

Strong personalities begin to share their vulnerabilities and fears.

Those who have always insisted on routine and structure try to be flexible and spontaneous.

The cold become more affectionate.

The meek show leadership.

The quiet speak up.

The angry attempt to forgive.

Trying to relate in new ways always stirs inner feelings of insecurity and fear of being rejected or misunderstood. If you notice your partner attempting to change in some basic way, react gently and nurturingly. Never criticize, ignore, or react with sarcasm or skepticism to a loved one's attempts to grow healthier.

Allowing Honest Reactions

Because of their healthy flexibility, families that cope positively with illness are able to tolerate a wide range of honest reactions from one another. Family members express a true and caring interest in how this illness and all its stresses are affecting other members. They ask one another questions, and they respond nurturingly to the answers, even if they do not have solutions.

When having such honest discussions, healthy families follow three basic rules of communication:

1. They use *"I" statements* in expressing feelings ("I feel safer when you take your blood pressure medicine regularly").

2. They avoid making *blaming statements* or accusing each other ("You're driving me crazy by not taking your medicine regularly").

3. They listen and let the speaker know what they have heard without reacting defensively.

Rule 3 can be called *nondefensive listening.* In the following example, Steven listens nondefensively to Alice's concerns, which allows Alice to respond nondefensively to Steven:

ALICE: I'm tired of monitoring what you eat. I worry about your diet, and I want you to take more responsibility for eating better. Sometimes I think I'm working harder at this than you are, and I end up feeling mad at you.

STEVEN: So you're feeling sort of tired and angry about keeping track of me?

ALICE: Yes, I am. It's a hard job.

STEVEN: I can hear your frustration, and I understand that this must get tiring. I know this is hard on you.

ALICE: Yes, it is.

STEVEN: I appreciate everything you do for me, and I don't mean to make you angry. I know you can't eat for me, and that it's my responsibility. I just have a hard time with this diet business.

ALICE: I feel for you. I know that all this change isn't easy. I just want you to know that I love you and that I'm concerned for you.

STEVEN: I do know that. And I love you.

Of course, such conversations do not always go this smoothly in real life. However, equipped with good communication tools and permission from family members to be open and honest, healthy families are able to resolve conflicts—even when family members strongly disagree. The key is that such families do not shame one another for any reason. They supportively allow one another to ventilate their feelings without trying to send the speaker on a guilt trip in return. They say out loud such things as the following:

"I'm sick and tired of all these trips to the doctor!"

"I know this has been hard on you, but I'm worn out, too."

"I couldn't sleep last night; I was afraid you might die."

"Sometimes I hold back telling you what's on my mind because I feel like I've already put you through too much agony."

When allowed such freedom to be open, people tend to be more honest and caring in dealing with each other. As they go through the process of rehabilitation, a man and a woman in a healthy relationship are especially likely to begin keeping tabs on each other's inner reactions. If you could secretly tape-record the private conversations of a healthy couple who are adjusting to illness, you might hear questions like the following being asked:

"Do you feel I understand you, in general?"

"Do you think I understand your feelings about _____?" (Fill in the blank with whatever you know to be a major concern of your spouse.)

"Do I respond to your feelings when you ask for support, or do I give you advice that sounds like an unsupportive lecture instead?"

"When I'm upset about something, am I clear in expressing to you what is on my mind, or do I simply act upset without being clear about what's bothering me?"

"When I'm upset, do I act like I blame you for my feelings?"

"When we disagree, do you feel that I deal with you fairly?"

"Are you worrying about things that you aren't talking with me about?"

"What are our kids saying to you about all this?"

"Does my surgery scar look disgusting to you?"

"Do I seem different to you since my surgery?"

No couple communicates perfectly, especially during emotional times. In healthy families, mistakes in communication are followed by apologies and by effective change in the communication process. By allowing one another the freedom to be honest in your family discussions, you can continue to grow together during this important time of changing relationships.

Getting the Right Information

Families who cope positively are forever curious about information relevant to what they are experiencing. Accurate information about heart illness and cardiac rehabilitation can soothe many anxieties and fears. Such information is almost always offered by medical personnel during the initial phases of treatment of heart illness, and more physicians and hospitals than ever before are now recognizing the need to include the patient's spouse in such educational programs.

However, my observation is that a cardiac couple's need for information outlives most physicians' availability to give information. Heart illness lasts a lifetime. What worked wonderfully during the first year of rehabilitation may not be so effective later. New concerns develop, and new information is needed to soothe these concerns.

Healthy cardiac couples select physicians who are willing to communicate with them in clear, compassionate, and respectful ways, and they use their own personal skills to maintain comfortable working relationships with these physicians. They respect themselves as having rights as patients, such as the right to information and the right to have one's spouse involved in consultations. They also realize that doctors are only human and have limits to their own levels of energy, patience, and skills.

You don't have to apologize for your need to continue asking questions about cardiac rehabilitation. But it is helpful, practical, and courteous to be respectful of your physician's busy schedule. Call and schedule an extended consultation with your doctor, indicating that you and your spouse have a number of questions that you would like addressed. In this way, the physician can plan time to spend with you. Do not ambush your doctor with twenty minutes of questions during what was scheduled as a ten-minute checkup.

Arrive at such consultations with a written list that will remind you of the questions you want addressed. Remember to say *Please* and *Thank you*. Both patients and doctors are people, and all people deserve to be dealt with in a caring fashion.

With these considerations in mind, remember these two main points: (1) You should find a doctor who is willing and able to take enough time to treat you with respect as a couple. Insist that your marriage, and not just one of your hearts, be recognized as a patient. (2) Take appropriate responsibility for your part of your care. Don't be a passive patient, waiting for some doctor to work magic in your life. In other words, remember to be assertive in finding out what you need to know about coping with this illness. Even more important, remember to put what you learn into practice:

Read about new low-cholesterol recipes and then try them out.

If you see an announcement of a lecture on modifying stress, attend, and try using what you learn.

Enroll in a class on meditation or relaxation and actually practice the exercises at home.

Join and participate in an organized cardiac rehabilitation program.

By gathering information, you can soothe your fears and develop an understanding of the realistic tasks involved in cardiac rehabilitation. This information goes a long way in preventing you from becoming bogged down in a nonproductive pit of questioning and guilt about why the illness happened.

Healthy couples have an interesting attitude toward the question What caused this illness? Their attitude is, "We don't care what caused it; we want to know what we have to do to recover." Rather than wallow in self-doubt and self-blame, these people demonstrate a process that I believe to be very adaptive when it comes to guilt management: *Guilt is a useful emotion if it is experienced for about three seconds and then leads to behavior change.*

Healthy couples accept that illness has entered their lives, and then they get about the task of making needed adjustments. They do not waste time moaning and groaning and living in confusion. They honestly look at their life-style and begin making the changes they need to ensure rehabilitation.

So decide realistically—with the help of professionals trained in cardiac rehabilitation and through your own assertive efforts—what you can do to recover, and then get to work as a healing team. Forget about *why;* focus on *how.* In this way, you can develop goals that give structure to your rehabilitation efforts.

Setting Goals

How many times have you decided to change some negative habit, only to fail in your efforts after a brief period of progress? This New Year's resolution syndrome—setting lofty goals that prove to be unattainable by about January 31—probably has much to do with the fact that the month of February brings with it the highest number of hospitalizations for treatment of depression.

Positive copers do not set themselves up for failure by committing to broad, all-encompassing, vaguely stated goals. Rather, they orchestrate their rehabilitation in a way that promotes feelings of success and continued motivation. They do this by setting concrete goals that are realistic, specific, and measurable, and then they often participate as a team in pursuing the goals. For example, they avoid setting vague goals such as "I will start getting more exercise." Instead, they set very specific goals: "We will walk for thirty minutes four times this week." Positive copers write these goals down and state them in a way that allows them to measure their own progress in tangible terms. By being specific in your goal setting, you can create an aura of cooperation and appreciation of each other: "Look at this exercise journal—I'm really proud of us. We both stuck to our plan this week."

The preceding example implies a point worth stating directly: Healthy couples do tend to participate in most aspects of cardiac rehabilitation together. This is good for the marriage, and it is also good for the heart patient. Numerous research studies have clearly shown that when spouses participate in the life-style changes that are suggested in cardiac rehabilitation, heart patients comply with the recommendations more closely. Healthy couples adopt a spirit of healthy living that begins to organize their family life as they go through the cardiac rehabilitation process together.

This does not mean that they always exercise at the same time, eat exactly the same meals, or take the same medicines. Further, this certainly does not mean that spouses are responsible for their mates' rehabilitation. But it does mean that healthy couples make rehabilitation a marital affair. The spouse turns the crisis of the illness into an opportunity to modify his or her own health habits in needed ways. In the process, cooperation and intimacy grow in the marriage.

By being specific and realistic in your goals, you can also avoid becoming demoralized and demotivated during the course of rehabilitation. Like heart illness itself, many of the positive cardiovascular effects of healthy life-style choices are invisible. There are, of course, exceptions to this statement: you can see your blood pressure readings improve, your cholesterol count drop, or your exercise tests improve.

However, these readings do not necessarily continue to change in positive directions, no matter how hard you work at rehabilitation. After all, no one—heart patient or otherwise—progresses in a straight line toward perfect physical conditioning, no matter how great the effort. If these are the only yardsticks being used to measure your success, then you may lose the motivation you need to continue your life-style changes.

Participants in our rehabilitation program at Wake Forest University go through a predictable pattern of motivation of this sort. Patients are given a treadmill test upon entering the program and then again every three months. Good improvement in exercise capacity is typical between the entry testing and the first follow-up testing. Motivation during the three-month period after the second testing is therefore predictably high; those black-and-white numbers from the testing show that healing is happening.

Then the trouble begins. Indicators of increased physical conditioning often begin to level off with the third treadmill test. This is perfectly normal in the rehabilitation course. In fact, a large percentage of healthy recovering patients periodically show slight declines in indicators of cardiac functioning during repeated treadmill tests. Motivation becomes even more difficult to maintain when the heart patient's rehabilitation is interfered with by further medical complications. Repeated heart attacks, need for bypass or "balloon" surgery, or increased angina may occur despite diligent efforts to overcome the effects of the original illness.

So how do you stay motivated even though those magic treadmill numbers or your own body may now be betraying your rehab efforts? Answer: Use tangible indicators of success in pursuing your rehabilitation goals.

Successfully recovering heart patients and their mates adopt the attitude that they will *live*—rather than die—with heart illness, and they accept that the illness will be part of the remaining years of their lives. They measure their rehabilitation progress in terms that are less dependent on medical scales and more easily tracked with honest self-monitoring. When they need a boost of motivation they ask themselves questions such as these:

Have I, indeed, exercised as regularly as I planned?

Have I made needed life-style changes like stopping smoking or limiting alcohol intake?

Am I eating a more heart-healthy diet?

Am I developing positive emotional and stress management habits?

Am I following my doctors' orders about medications?

If you have done a reasonable (not perfect, but *reasonable*) job in these regards, then you deserve to pat yourself on the back with a tangible reward, regardless of what the treadmill, the blood analysis, or any other medical test indicates. I do not mean to imply that these test results are unimportant. On the contrary, be realistic in dealing with the implications of such tests. It may be that you have to change your rehabilitation plan, based on the hard medical facts. The point is that *positive copers motivate themselves by making note of what they are doing well and by rewarding themselves accordingly.* Healthy couples help each other remain motivated throughout rehabilitation by giving nurturing and appreciative feedback to each other. Each takes note of what the other does that is right and good. They make lists of the many positive health care choices they make regularly, and they skip shaming and fussing about each other's imperfections.

Taking appropriate care of yourself is easier if you are supported in your efforts by caring attention from others. Healthy families seem to know this, and they treat each other in this spirit.

Coming to Peace

Why do bad things happen to good people? This is the question examined in a popular book of similar title, and it is the question that is asked on a personal level by most people affected by heart disease. Patients and families who heal tend to be people who come to some form of psychological and spiritual peace about the fact that this illness has happened, and about the meaning of their lives now that they are dealing with rehabilitation.

Healthy couples often soothe many of their fears by turning to their belief in some Higher Power. This might be (and most often is) belief in a nurturing God. For some, this soothing and its accompanying motivation to recover come from the power of belief in family and the desire to improve intimate connections. Regardless of the form this Higher Power takes, I have seldom encountered a successfully recovered family who did not have some such belief system. Through such beliefs, these families are better able to make sense of their suffering. They find a higher level of meaning to their life together and a new motivation to live in more loving connection with one another. The power and maturity of these perspectives help such families strengthen their love for one another while healing together.

Finally, even though illness has become a factor in their lives, healthy families are able to continue growing and changing in all the normal ways families grow and change. Every family tends to freeze when crisis hits. Major decisions to move on in development are put on hold until the crisis passes. In dealing with chronic illness, some families never redecide this rule to freeze. Everyone's development then suffers. As in the case of the Hinson family, this decision not to go on with life might be made either consciously or unconsciously. The son in the Hinson family was not told out loud by his mother any of the following: "Lose your fiancée"; "Stop developing a life of your own outside this family"; "Freeze!"; or "Come home and live miserably ever after." The Hinson son was not told any of these messages; he just "heard" them in his natural reaction to his father's illness and to his mother's despair.

Members of the healthy couple explicitly give each other and other family members permission to go on with life, even though one of them now has heart illness. Children are encouraged to continue to grow up, leave home, establish their careers, and raise their own families. Vacations are still taken and enjoyed. A spouse's plans to return to school, take up new hobbies, make new friends—or whatever signals an ongoing living of life—all continue. Make cardiac rehabilitation an important *part of,* but *not all of* your life together.

Summary

Even healthy families react to illness in ways that show that coping with illness is an evolving process, not a single event. Families do not automatically get this adjustment "right" and then go on from there. Rather, they are forever having to readjust, modify, and reevaluate their coping strategies.

However, healthy families adjust to illness not only by surviving but by actually improving the overall quality of their relations with one another. Following the stress and distress experienced during the initial and intermediate stages of adjustment, healthy families begin to reorganize relatively quickly.

The shock of the illness often results in family members reevaluating their relationships with one another. In the light of this honest look into the mirror of the family, they renew their appreciation of and commitments to one another. Such positive reactions will occur in your family if you relate to each other in ways that

- maintain communication and organization within the family;
- promote independence and self-esteem for each member;
- maintain family bonds and family unity;
- encourage role change and flexibility;
- maintain social supports and outside-the-family activities; and
- control the impact of stress so that the family does not lose its organization.

In going through this adjustment, you must avoid the many family potholes that mar the road to recovery. The major family pitfalls to avoid are discussed in the next chapter.

Five

Pitfalls of Family Life

. . . . . .

When a heart patient is not coping well with illness, the signs are usually obvious. Depression, failure to comply with medical recommendations, persistent irritability and worry, all send clear messages to everyone in the family that poor adjustment is in progress. The signs that a family is coping poorly are not always obvious, however. The web of family problems within which a heart patient sometimes gets caught is often deathly silent. I have worked with many families in which the heart patient is coping quite well but is worried constantly about the inner struggles of the spouse or the children.

Remember, *families always react as teams*. Tension floating around within a family may erupt in symptoms at any spot in the family. This might translate into troubling reactions by individual family members or into tension within certain family relationships.

Signs of Poor Family Coping

How can you tell how well you and your loved ones are coping with this illness? To begin with, you might examine the following nine signs of poor adjustment, and carefully consider whether your family is experiencing any of these difficulties.

40

1. *Depression.* Grief is a normal and healthy reaction to illness. While grieving, a family member may be sad and irritable, may cry frequently, may have insomnia, and may be preoccupied with rehabilitation concerns. Such grieving usually passes within several months as the reality of the illness settles in and motivation to rehabilitate begins to grow. However, some family members react to illness by becoming seriously depressed—a condition that paralyzes rehabilitation and family life in ways that grieving does not. Although grief and depression may look and feel similar in many ways, important differences between these two conditions do exist.

Grief is time limited; depression is not. When a person is depressed, feelings of sadness may never lift for any length of time. Depressed people feel stuck in repetitive thoughts and feelings that are frightening and painful. These often include thoughts of death or suicide. Guilt, anxiety, or anger may fill every moment for a depressed person. Constant worry and distress may lead to sleep problems, physical aches and pains, mood changes, or preoccupation with thoughts of death or suicide.

Unlike grief, depression is not relieved by talking with others. For some people, depression leads to complete emotional and physical shutdown: no more tears come; ability to function is severely compromised; concentration and ability to think become fuzzy; interest in life and ability to experience pleasure seem lost forever.

It is essential to understand that clinical depression of this sort is a *medical* condition that requires appropriate treatment. No amount of pep talks, positive thinking, or messages like "Pull yourself up by your bootstraps and get on with life" will cure clinical depression. Most clinically depressed people require both medication and professional psychological help to overcome this condition.

The good news is that not only can depression be treated—it can be cured. Typical reactions to current psychological, medical, and psychiatric treatments for depression fall into the category of modern medical miracles. Help is available. If any member of your family persists in showing the symptoms just described *for more than eight weeks,* help that loved one to seek appropriate treatment.

2. *Failure to accept the diagnosis.* Some families never say the *H*-word out loud; they never openly talk about the fact that a member of

the family has heart illness. One such family whom I treated insisted on referring to their mother's angina as "upset stomach." Others constantly change doctors, searching for one who will participate in their denial. Still others refuse to accept the need for taking rehabilitation seriously and make statements such as "High blood pressure just runs in our family, and no one has died young yet. It's nothing to worry about."

3. *Denying the symptoms of illness.* One relative of mine who recently underwent quadruple coronary artery bypass surgery after his first visit to a cardiologist admitted that for years he had been experiencing crushing chest pains whenever he walked in the woods on cold days in hunting season. Rather than accept these pains as a sign of illness, he reported that he would usually just sit beneath a tree and pound his chest until the pain stopped. Now, *that's* denial!

4. *Remaining ignorant about the illness.* Unhealthy families refuse to learn the details of heart illness and cardiac rehabilitation. This refusal often signifies a passive, victimized attitude in reaction to the illness, an attitude that will surely work against successful adjustment.

5. *Flights into activity.* Some patients and families react to illness by running—not as in *exercising*; as in *scared to death*. They act as though they fear that life is almost over and that they therefore need to cram as much as possible into their remaining days. The result might be impulsive behavior that just makes life more complicated. For others, the flight into activity happens as part of staying stuck in the bargaining stage of grieving. These people believe, "If I try hard enough and behave perfectly enough, then this illness will disappear." This belief might lead to trying as many different rehabilitation strategies as possible, all in the shortest possible period of time; shopping for magical cures; doubling exercise or dietary changes; or engaging in superstitious behaviors.

These frantic flights into activity can be mistaken for indications of a positive attitude. In reality, such hyperactivity can lead people to take unhealthy risks and to disconnect from others because they are obsessively focusing on all this action.

Disconnecting from other people by focusing on activity is a way some families defend against fears of becoming emotionally close with the sick loved one. Many families live in fear that the heart patient will die, and they begin preparing themselves for this death as soon as illness hits. Unfortunately, such families sometimes stay stuck in the habit of keeping their distance even though the patient outlives everyone else in the family!

6. *Persistent hostility.* Many people are angry long before their lives are affected by heart disease. These people simply become even more hostile in response to the stresses of illness. Their typical grouchiness escalates to the point of losing emotional control in reaction to minor irritants. For other people, however, irritability, moodiness, snappiness, and temper tantrums seem to add up to a personality change. Many such people are stuck in the anger stage of grief and are failing to progress toward accepting their current reality. It is as though their anger is an expression of the desperate cry "I don't want to have to deal with this!"

Any family member can become stuck in this syndrome. Families sometimes cooperate in fueling anger by collectively targeting their hostilities toward medical personnel. The pattern is often obvious. It may also be expressed quite indirectly, as in the case of Erin and her family.

Erin was a soft-spoken woman who kept her emotional reactions private. In the months following her bypass surgery, she remained pleasant in her dealings with friends and extended family. But Erin and her husband were seethingly angry over their frustrated efforts to get what they considered reasonable medical care. This was this couple's arena of quiet—and risky—rebellion against illness.

With the support and encouragement of her husband, Erin repeatedly changed cardiologists. She pitted doctors against each other, telling one half-truths about the advice she had been given by another. She stalked out of waiting rooms never to return if she was kept waiting more than twenty minutes beyond her scheduled appointment time. All this was done to the applause of her spouse. As a result of this behavior, Erin and her husband were left quietly enraged and without any consistent medical care. No one knew of their rage. It was their secret way of distracting themselves from their pain.

7. *Prolonged exaggeration of typical personality traits.* Anger is not the only coping reaction that may become exaggerated in a family's efforts

to manage the impact of illness. Any outstanding personality characteristics of any family member may become magnified when people are coping with scary levels of stress.

The orderly individual may become compulsive about routines and details. The grouchy family member may become sullen and openly hostile. The suspicious, skeptical person may become over cautious to the point of appearing paranoid. The low-energy homebody may become withdrawn and depressed. The person who often complained of various aches and pains may become preoccupied with symptoms of physical illness. The generally gloomy, pessimistic individual may become paralyzed by fear of death.

Such alarm reactions may be temporary responses to the shock of illness. But these patterns should calm down and the individual should return to normal personality patterns within four to six months of the onset of the stressful event. By that time, the disorientation and shock of reacting to illness typically lift. Continued exaggeration of coping style beyond this period may suggest the need for more open discussion and counseling from family minister, doctor, or therapist.

8. *Discounting the possibility of coping.* Some families have the attitude that coping with heart illness is impossible. Their passive acceptance of illness can lead to many unhealthy choices, such as the following:

- Refusal to accept referral for help with physical or psychological aspects of rehabilitation.

- No expression of interest in learning about the illness or the rehabilitation strategies.

- Repeatedly "forgetting about" or openly refusing to attend medical follow-up appointments.

- Subtly or openly refusing to participate in attempts to change long-held family traditions (such as eating unhealthily) that work against rehabilitation.

9. *Children or teenagers showing signs of distress.* Most children equate having a heart attack with dying. The idea of losing a parent is terrifying for children of any age. Unfortunately, children also tend to have difficulty expressing their feelings, and parents tend to fear that talking openly with children about upsetting topics will only frighten

them. These factors combine in many families, with the result that children hold in a storm of emotions—fear, anger, grief, embarrassment, guilt—in reaction to a parent's illness. These unsoothed feelings can lead to various signs of struggle, depending on the child's age:

- Decline in school performance.
- Eating or sleeping problems.
- Frequent nightmares.
- Behavioral problems.
- Outbursts of temper.
- Vague or persistent physical problems.
- Fears of being alone with the heart patient.
- Clinginess.
- Excessive withdrawal or tiredness.
- Drug or alcohol use.
- Excessive efforts to please or to "be good."
- Oppositional, rebellious behavior.
- Refusal to discuss problems, especially feelings about heart illness.

It is important to help children cope with a parent's illness. Begin by talking with them about how you are reacting to your own fears and frustrations. Letting them see your struggle will help them feel more normal and will model for them how to express their own struggles more openly. Ask if they have questions about what is happening or what will happen now that your family is coping with illness. If they have no questions, give them information anyway. They may listen more than they let you know. Give them information that is appropriate to their age and that conveys hope and confidence that your family will endure this chapter of your life. It is okay to admit that you don't know all the answers, especially to hard questions like "Is Daddy going to die from this heart attack?"

At the same time, it is important to reassure your children that you are receiving good medical care and that you will continue to do all you can to recover. You might consider offering to arrange for children, especially teenagers, to talk with someone other than you and your spouse about their reactions. Brief counseling—either individual or family counseling—can be tremendously helpful to children who are struggling with major changes in family life. It is helpful to inform school guidance counselors that your family is going through a crisis. The counselor can share this information with the child's teachers.

As your rehabilitation progresses, talk openly and frequently about cardiac rehabilitation being a family affair. Regularly hold family meetings during which you encourage open discussion of your reactions to this illness or to one another. You need to be the role models, demonstrating that talking openly is beneficial to the whole family. Ask the children questions: How are they reacting to the new foods everyone is eating and to the changes that have occurred in your exercise and stress management habits? Encourage everyone to express concerns about one another. Find out what you need from one another to help make the coming week more comfortable. And be sure to point out what you have noticed and appreciated about one another during the past week.

It is especially important to let all children know that they had nothing to do with the parent's illness. Children are self-centered in their insecurities, and they need explicit reassurance that their behavior did not cause the illness. Further, let them know that you—both parents—will help them and each other to cope. Reassure your children that you do not need them to take care of you.

These nine signs of poor coping by no means exhaust the ways families may signal unhealthy reactions to the stress of illness. In fact, symptoms of poor coping may not be related in any obvious way to the impact of illness on the family. For example, grown children in a cardiac family may begin experiencing their own symptoms: emotional problems, physical illness, or career or marital struggles. Or the heart patient's spouse may begin to experience new health problems or flare-ups of old problems that everyone thought had disappeared.

What causes such family-related problems in coping? Perhaps the troubled family member simply needs more attention and reassurance during this frightening time. Gently confronting the family member—describing the behavior that is concerning you, and stressing your

concern and love for that person and your willingness to be of help—
is certainly the first move to make.

However, such direct invitations to talk about what is troubling
someone do not always bear the fruit of resolving the obvious problems. Why does open communication not always work in solving such
problems? The answer lies in the often subtle ways families may shift
unhealthily as the stress of illness stretches them beyond their coping
point.

Changes in Family Dynamics Following Illness

Families coping with illness are at risk of encountering a wide variety
of problems. For some families, the stress of rehabilitation makes old
relationship problems worse. Other families develop unhealthy solutions to their fears for one another about the anticipated impact of illness; or they may become involved in unhealthy struggles with one
another in the aftershock of illness. No matter how loving or healthy
your family may be, the stress of illness heightens your risk of developing unhealthy relationship patterns.

Before describing the various troublesome family reactions to illness that should be guarded against, I want to stress that *problems in a
family are seldom due to a single cause, and a given family problem seldom
has a single effect.*

A complex medical-behavioral-emotional-family event such as a
heart attack taxes any family's ability to remain reasonably organized.
It is my opinion that every family goes through phases in which some
of the following problem modes of relating occur. The crucial issue in
evaluating how well you are adjusting as a family is the extent to
which these patterns persist despite your efforts to adapt.

Dancing Harder Than Ever: Old Problems Get Worse

The longer I practice clinical psychology, the more amazed I am to observe that families, like individuals, tend to know what they are doing

that contributes to their problems, but they continue to do it harder and harder the more frustrated and frightened they become. Many families coping with heart illness react this way. Now that they are threatened by overwhelming illness-related stress, they exaggerate family roles that were not working very well in the first place. Two such family patterns are (1) amplifying typical family roles and (2) exaggerating existing differences in perceptions.

Amplifying Family Roles under Stress

Another contribution of the family therapist Virginia Satir was her notion that family members tend to assume certain roles to maintain balance in overall family functioning. Four primary roles are assigned and assumed in family life, and these roles become exaggerated during stressful times. The four roles can be seen at work in families with more or fewer than four members, too: family members often trade off roles.

1. The first role is that of trying to soothe others by *running interference* for the family and by being especially attentive to the needs and feelings of other family members. People playing this role agree with others in order to avoid conflict and even apologize when they are in the right if conflict does occur. In dealing with any prolonged family stress event, these folks are prone to assume the role of martyr within the family. They put their own needs so far aside that they end up feeling deprived and unappreciated.

2. The second role is *finding fault* in what others do, especially during times of high stress. The faultfinder responds to internal discomfort and fear by conveying a specific message to other people: "If it weren't for you, everything would be okay." Needless to say, people who are invested in keeping everything on an even keel—people playing the running interference role described above—are particularly susceptible to the guilt induced by being blamed for a loved one's discomfort.

3. People in the third role react to stress by *being extremely unemotional.* These people have difficulty initiating and responding to emotional communications within the family. The more emotion floating around the family, the more reasonable, data oriented, and unfeeling such people act.

4. People fill the fourth role by *drawing attention away from the family's pain.* The words and actions of these people often seem irrelevant to what is happening at the moment. Sometimes these people call attention to themselves by developing a life crisis or a health problem. The effect of such behavior is the temporary alleviation of the family's pain and distress over some more frightening stressor—such as heart illness.

When the family stress and fear levels escalate, exaggerated interplay among these roles can occur. In reacting to the stresses of heart illness, many couples get stuck in a dance in which one finds fault with everything and the other spends all his or her energy trying to soothe the first person's feelings. The heart patient may take on the first role, reacting to issues having to do with the illness by telling his or her partner, "My cholesterol levels are still too high! If you'd learn to cook healthier meals, maybe I'd live longer." The partner is often all too familiar with his or her own role and readily settles into feeling anxious and guilty about the spouse's rehabilitation struggles. The partner's steps in this dance involve remaining quiet about his or her own needs and trying to avoid further blame by pleasing the other person. Remembering that reactions within families fuel counterreactions, you should not be surprised to find that such a couple soon gets stuck in a circular dance: the more one person complains, the more the other placates, and so on.

As tensions mount in the marriage, the whole family team may heat up in emotional reactions. Other family members may react to the tension of this dance by exaggerating their own typical family positions. For example, a child might try to divert attention from this scary process by misbehaving. This distracting behavior might fuel an overrational response by the family member who always keeps cool. In an effort to counterbalance the child's failure to attend to the main issues at hand, this family member may become progressively more rational and logical in reacting to the emotional situation. Such people often appear cold to others, but in fact they are typically concerned and lonely behind the walls of all of that logic.

The more emotional tension mounts in the family, the more these pre-illness family roles escalate by fueling one another. Thus, many families settle into patterns of reacting to illness that simply make matters worse.

Disagreeing about the Illness—and about Everything Else

The second unhealthy relationship pattern that can become exaggerated in reaction to illness is the habit of always disagreeing. Some couples seem locked into this habit. She says it's sunny, he says it's cloudy. She feels hot, he feels cold. He's ready to kiss and make up, she's still angry. This pattern of disagreeing is often based on true differences of perspective, but it is sometimes fueled by failure to resolve underlying relationship issues that have left a sense of distrust and resentment in the relationship. The constant disagreeing becomes a way of expressing underlying negative feelings.

Some couples, like Jim and Peggy, take this habit to the point of disagreeing about the very existence of illness.

Jim was a very emotional, dramatic individual who perpetually complained that his wife, Peggy, should show him more love and attention. He frequently complained to Peggy, "Just because I'm a man, it doesn't mean I don't feel fear and need reassurance."

Peggy was disgusted and angry with Jim over his "constant whining" and over the many times in their marriage when she had been manipulated by him. She was especially angry about an extramarital affair that Jim had had many years ago with someone from whom he was supposedly getting medical help with one of his many vague health problems.

Jim had a moderately serious heart attack one year before I met him and Peggy. They were referred by Jim's cardiologist, who was concerned about Peggy's refusal to accept the reality of her husband's heart condition. She adamantly refused to participate in any cardiac rehabilitation efforts. The cardiologist was also puzzled by Jim's tendency to exaggerate his physical symptoms. From a medical perspective, he was in reasonably good shape now, but he continued to show up for appointments with a wealth of complaints and lists of vague symptoms.

As I got to know this couple, it became apparent that they were locked in a dance revolving around Jim's health concerns. Their dialogue about Jim's condition was symbolic of their long-term struggles with intimacy and trust. Jim now requested attention and special consideration from Peggy by acting as though he might die any minute. Peggy expressed her distrust and anger toward Jim by openly doubting that he had even had a heart attack.

Whenever Jim complained of having chest pains, Peggy chided him, saying, "You're not going to fool me like you did those doctors; I know you, and they don't. Everybody has chest pains sometimes. That's not the same as having a heart attack. You just need to grow up and stop expecting to always get your way in life."

The more Peggy criticized and withheld affection, the more Jim complained about his health; the more Jim complained about his health, the more Peggy criticized rather than nurtured; and so on. Jim and Peggy were stuck in a relationship cycle that fueled illness behavior. But this dance also allowed them to interact around a topic (Jim's illness) that was in many ways less painful and complicated for them than the underlying marital issue of lost trust and intimacy.

Even couples who are not as seriously troubled as Jim and Peggy are likely to disagree in their reactions to heart illness and cardiac rehabilitation. Unlike many other disabilities, such as having a leg amputated, heart illness has invisible effects. It is therefore easy for a couple to adopt different notions about the seriousness of the illness or the extent to which the patient's activities and roles need to be changed because of the illness.

Furthermore, some couples simply differ in their overall attitude toward life: one feels that we are Born to Choose in reacting to life, and the other feels that we are Born to Lose. In this same vein, the couple may adopt different philosophies in reacting to illness. These philosophies then shape an attitude that affects the different ways each individual reacts to the illness on a day-to-day basis. Illness may be viewed in various ways:

- As a *challenge*—a life situation that consists of multiple tasks that must be mastered.
- As an *enemy*, like an invasion of harmful forces that have entered your life and body.
- As a *punishment* being delivered justly or unjustly for your lack of perfection.
- As a sign of *weakness*.
- As a *relief* from your typical life stresses.
- As a *strategy* to use in trying to get more nurturing attention from the world.
- As a *irreparable loss* of valuable aspects of life.
- As an *opportunity* for growth and development.

Differences between partners in their reactions to the meaning of illness almost always lead to increased conflict during rehabilitation. For example, suppose one spouse views the illness as a challenge to be overcome, and the other sees it as an excuse to slow down and be less goal oriented. Such a couple is likely to define the very tasks necessary for rehabilitation quite differently. The first spouse will approach rehabilitation by working hard to change various cardiac risk factors. The second spouse will define success in rehabilitation as learning to take it easy and not be so serious about any rat race—including the need to change cardiac risk factors.

If you and your mate seem stuck in differing views of the meaning of heart illness and its impact on your life, it may be helpful for you to pinpoint the specific thinking patterns that underlie your differences in perspective. To do this, you must honestly evaluate whether this disagreement is a symptom of unforgiven hurts or unresolved problems in other areas of your relationship.

Unhealthy family patterns—amplifying stress positions and exaggerating differences of perspective—obviously interfere with both family intimacy and cardiac rehabilitation. These patterns sometimes combine with the following family pitfalls to complicate the rehabilitation process even more.

The Family Scramble

As is evident by now, I strongly believe that few events in life create as much of a scramble in family functioning as heart illness. Families coping with illness get pushed to the point of losing the organization that holds them together. This family scramble is heightened if the "wrong" family member gets sick or if the illness hits a marriage that is already caught in a painful struggle over intimacy.

The Wrong Person Got Sick!

No family wants any of its members to get sick, but we have less difficulty coping with illness if it strikes a member who is already defined as being the "sickly one" or the "weak one" or the "problem" in the family.

For example, a family may have grown accustomed to dealing with the health problems caused by the husband's alcoholism. If he now has a heart attack, the specific problems change, but the processes of living with a husband who has a health problem simply continue. The family may already be used to coping with the husband's illness when the heart attack happens, and the shock of this illness may therefore be less than if he had never been sick before.

On the other hand, this family would have more difficulty coping if the wife were to get sick. Then the family member who had been the primary caretaker of the family (because of her husband's alcoholism) would be temporarily unavailable to hold the family together in the face of escalating stress. Family adjustment to this illness would be understandably more difficult.

Such family scrambles in adjustment occur not only in reaction to the family caretaker's illness. Any time the impact of illness requires family members to make major shifts in their modes of relating to one another, the family is at risk of developing adjustment problems. Families who are shocked by illness struggle to remain organized in familiar ways. In their efforts to help one another maintain comfortable and familiar roles within the family, some families make the unhealthy choice of either denying that the illness exists or having someone in the family "one-downing" the heart patient by becoming even more symptomatic than the patient.

Pretending Nothing Has Happened

Heart patients and their families sometimes cooperate in denying that anyone in the family has heart disease; they seem to be playing a game of pretending that the illness is not real. This might lead to the nine signs of poor family coping described earlier in this chapter. In my experience, it is a mistake to assume that patients who deny illness are necessarily afraid of being sick. Although they often are, denial of illness frequently has more to do with the patient's fear of the impact that open acknowledgment of the illness will have on loved ones. Mr. Russo was an example.

Mr. Russo was the elderly, powerful patriarch of a close-knit family. He had lived much of his life accepting the role of protecting his wife from worries in order to help her cope with her tendency to suffer bouts of depression. When this man had a massive heart attack, he refused to implement cardiac rehabilitation recommendations. Whenever he was confronted by his doctor for his failure to begin exercising or stop smoking, Mr. Russo would simply say, "I'm not the only one to consider here."

This patient's reaction to his illness was certainly unhealthy from a medical standpoint, but his reaction made sense according to the unique logic of family teamwork. He denied his illness rather than force his wife to remember that he was sick. He did not have undue fears for himself; he was protecting his wife, just as he always had.

Getting Sicker Than the Patient

Another pattern of family scramble that results when the "wrong" family member gets sick involves a spouse making a sacrifice to protect the patient's self-esteem. In this pattern, the spouse who is not the heart patient develops symptoms that allow the heart patient to maintain a sense of importance and power in the family despite the presence of the illness.

Research has suggested that more than 50 percent of family members of heart patients develop psychosomatic ailments that require medical attention. Many of these ailments result from the sheer stress of coping with having a sick loved one. I believe the desire to protect each other is another factor that often underlies this reaction. Joseph and Toni were stuck in such a pattern.

Like many traditional couples, Joseph and Toni had organized their marriage and family around the understanding that Joseph was the head of the household. He was the strong leader in the family. He worked hard in his career, and he provided well for everyone. He was the voice of calm and guidance during times of family crisis and stress. He was the rock of stability upon which the family was built and functioned.

No one had planned on Joseph's developing severe hardening of the arteries and requiring quadruple bypass surgery at age fifty-five. Even less planned was this formerly strong man's subsequent loss of self-confidence and his development of paralyzing depression. He withdrew from friends and business associates, and he began doubting himself so severely that he began to have problems in his career. He even became unsure of his opinions in reacting to normal family decisions that fill day-to-day life.

Joseph's depression and coping paralysis began to improve however, when Toni began to develop symptoms of illness. She began experiencing anxiety attacks whenever she left the house. She also became obsessed with worry about her parents' failing health and was overwhelmed with trying to figure out how to help them.

As his wife's functioning deteriorated even further than his own, Joseph seemed to regain his sense of self as a strong and important person who was needed to protect and provide for his loved ones. His depression lifted, and his overall capacity for functioning in a healthy manner improved. After all, he had to help his poor, ailing wife.

These family patterns of denial and of one-downing the sick member demonstrate that symptoms in a family (such as denial of illness, or psychosomatic reactions) often serve as a solution to an underlying family problem. As painful as these symptoms may be, they may hurt less than the alternative: watching a loved one grope in pain.

Indirect Battles for Power

Unhealthy couples have difficulty with intimacy. When the stress of illness and recovery is added to their struggles, they often resort to indirect ways of battling with each other. These indirect strategies can create yet another version of the family scramble to remain organized, and they can complicate cardiac rehabilitation.

The basic problem in some marriages is that one or both partners do not respond to direct, open, and honest requests for behavior change. For example, an unhealthy partner has trouble responding to direct feedback such as, "I feel lonely when you don't talk with me. I'd like you to notice me more, ask me about my days, and be more affectionate with me." Or "Sometimes I just like to be quiet and into my own thoughts and hobbies. It's not that I'm angry or want to shut you out; it's just that I sometimes want my own space."

When partners fail in their attempts to negotiate needed change in their marriage openly, indirect struggles to change each other often result. Two such indirect attempts to change the relationship are (1) assuming a helpless or passive position in the marriage and (2) developing a chronic symptom.

Passive Power

Being passive can be a very powerful way to control a relationship. I often see couples in which one member seems to wield all the power by being the decision maker, the spokesperson for the family (and for the spouse's thoughts and feelings), and the orchestrator of the family activities. However, such marriages often have a secret: the seemingly powerless, passive spouse is actually in control. The passive one controls the brakes in the system. The relationship does not move unless the passive one cooperates, no matter how forcefully the "powerful" spouse mashes the relationship accelerator.

Signs of a couple struggling in this way might be the passive spouse's refusal to get excited—about a trip that the powerhouse has scheduled, about the guests the powerhouse has invited over for dinner, or about sex. In the example of sexual passivity, the message to the overbearing spouse is often quite obvious: "You may be able to control our life and outtalk me and convince me that my thoughts and feelings don't make sense, but you can't turn me on sexually."

Now, who do you think has the power in such a relationship?

Unfortunately, such passive power maneuvering can seriously interfere with recovery from heart illness. When passive spouses get sick, they usually treat the tasks of cardiac rehabilitation with the same passivity that characterizes their participation in the marriage. Such patients tend to settle into a sick role that further justifies their passive style of manipulating the marriage. Although they may quietly win their marital struggles, they may lose their lives by failing to recover from heart illness.

The Power of Symptoms

Some people get caught in the trap of exaggerating their physical symptoms in reaction to relationship problems. They do not do so consciously; they simply feel stuck and miserable. Their health is poor, and their family life is worse. This unhealthy relationship pattern does not always revolve around symptoms of heart disease. I have worked with cardiac couples who dance no dysfunctional dances around the cardiac rehabilitation process but instead play out their power struggle around one spouse's sexual performance problems or the other spouse's arthritis, or alcoholism, or preoccupation over their children. The content doesn't matter. The process of being symptomatic in a way that controls the relationship is the point of this marital pattern.

Furthermore, this form of marital struggle does not always involve the passive spouse developing an illness. A variation of this same relationship dance involves the less obviously powerful mate's reaction to the powerful mate's heart illness.

As is shown by the case of Tom and Lena, although certain reactions on the part of the "weaker" spouse increase his or her power within the marriage, these same reactions can significantly complicate the ill spouse's course of medical rehabilitation. This case also demonstrates the complex interplay in which both spouses indirectly use physical symptoms in an attempt to resolve marital struggles.

Tom was a classic Type A personality: hard driving, competitive, excessively focused on work, and seemingly unbothered by the stresses of his life. Like many such men, Tom was also rather uncomfortable with the whole realm of intimacy and was driven by the insecurities that lurked beneath the surface of his powerful style.

For years, Tom and his wife, Lena, had struggled with his tendency to ignore marriage and family life. Lena often became fed up with Tom's refusal to change and separated from him briefly twice, only to return home and continue the frustrating marriage. After twenty-six years of marriage, Lena had all but given up hope that Tom would ever slow down and attend to her and to their children. Then, with no prior warnings of failing health, Tom had a heart attack at the age of fifty-three.

By the time of Tom's heart attack, he and Lena had settled into a life of lonely frustration and extreme stress. Each of them lived in fear of the other's outbursts of anger and blaming modes of communicating. Tension was escalating to the point of another marital separation when Tom's heart attack stopped them in their tracks.

The heart attack gave Tom and Lena a new arena in which to play out their relationship struggles and their individual psychological issues. Lena now had a new power lever for getting her husband to respond to her needs—the doctors: "The doctors all say you need to slow down, relax, eat your meals at home, attend your kids' ball games, and generally start to enjoy life. So don't tell me I'm just whining when I fuss at you about these things!"

Tom, too, now had an indirect way of handling his own emotional pain. He had always harbored secret fears of his own stress levels and of the demands to perform that he had created with his own career momentum. He often wanted more soothing intimacy with his family, but he always had difficulty asking directly for such closeness. Now his heart illness had provided him with a less embarrassing and more comfortable way of getting his family to meet his needs for nurturing and intimacy. He now had a medically justified reason to slow down and enjoy life more. As long as he stayed sick, life would feel more comfortable and his wife and children would seem closer to him.

Summary

Each of the family pitfalls described in this chapter can cause serious problems in families and can seriously interfere with the cardiac rehabilitation process. If you and your family are caught in any of the coping pitfalls described in this chapter, it is important to be realistic about this fact: You risk sabotaging cardiac rehabilitation efforts if you do not correct these problems.

What can be done? In general, you must work together to strengthen your marriage by learning to be more intimate and helpful to each other in managing yourselves and the stresses of the rehabilitation process. The remainder of this book outlines specific ways to accomplish these important tasks. We will begin with a discussion of the most neglected topic in cardiac rehabilitation: how adult children of heart patients are affected by a parent's illness, and how such children can free their parents to heal together.

Six

Adult Children of Heart Patients

■　■　■　■　■

The adult children of heart patients are perhaps the best hidden of all the victims of heart illness. The majority of heart patients in the United States have adult children, most of whom live within a two-hour drive of their parents.

Many of these grown children become the primary emotional (and, often, physical) caretakers of their parents as the parents begin dealing with the debilitating effects of aging or illness. As a result, many grown children become caught in a web of family stress during that in-between stage of life that involves attempting to create a new family and career while trying at the same time to remain loyal and loving to one's first family.

Remaining lovingly connected with one's family throughout life is certainly a healthy—and a recommended—way of living. So why all this talk about adult children as "victims" of the stress of heart illness? The unfortunate truth is that many adult children do not *choose* to be lovingly connected with their aging parents; they feel compelled to do so out of some deep sense of guilt and concern. These uncomfortable feelings often fuel poor choice making for the children, resulting in their becoming involved with their original family in ways that actually interfere with their own adult lives. Furthermore, this involvement by adult children in their parents' struggles may help cover up problems within the parents' relationship that need to be addressed.

Marital Tensions and Adult Children

In chapter 5, various family pitfalls in coping with illness were discussed. Examples were given of the unhealthy pattern of couples in conflict choosing to focus on illness as a means of avoiding their differences. By focusing on a shared problem, such as one partner's illness, a couple in marital trouble can temporarily avoid facing problems that are brewing in their relationship—problems that may frighten them more than the illness does.

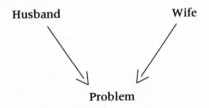

Perhaps even more common in such situations is the family pattern of reducing the anxiety and tension that are mounting in a relationship by focusing on a third party. Family therapists call this family pattern *triangulation,* because the pattern of relating can be depicted as a triangle:

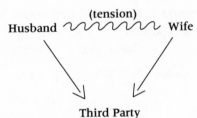

Triangulation seems to be an inevitable characteristic of human relationships. As tension mounts between two people, they tend to draw a third party into their relationship mess. This process is seen in all relationships, not only in families coping with illness. For example, two coworkers get into conflict and each begins gossiping about the other to a third party. Unfortunately, when this process occurs in families the couple in conflict usually triangulates one of their children. The consequence may be that the child begins to feel closer to one parent at the expense of the relationship with the other parent:

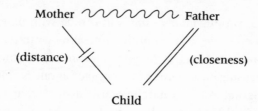

In this pattern, a child may begin to side with and soothe one parent and, in so doing, become distanced from the other parent. In families coping with heart illness, an adult child may support the heart patient parent who is complaining of being mistreated or misunderstood by the other parent. Or the adult child may side with the spouse of the heart patient, trying secretly to soothe that parent's anxieties and fears about the impact of the cardiac rehabilitation process on the marriage. In either case, the adult child develops closeness with one parent at the expense of closeness with the other parent—a situation that is guaranteed to distress any child.

Some children become counselors to both parents. Each parent turns to one or more of the grown offspring rather than to each other for soothing of the pains caused by the illness or by tensions that have developed in the marriage. Out of well-intentioned love and concern, the children offer their parents encouragement and "parental" advice on how to deal with the problems that are affecting the marriage.

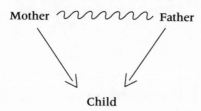

The Cost of Triangles

Triangles between friends and co-workers can be trouble, but triangles within a family are *always* trouble. It is always painful for one family member to be caught in a conflict between two loved ones. Regardless of the ages of the children in a family, they are vulnerable to and negatively affected by being drawn into their parents' relationship difficulties.

Triangulation in families causes many problems. First, triangulation interferes with the couple's ability to resolve their differences; distracting themselves by turning to a child for comfort provides only temporary relief as the relationship problems increase.

Second, any family member suffers marked physical and psychological alarm when placed in a position of conflicting loyalties between two loved ones. This fact may contribute to the high incidence of stress-related disorders in families coping with illness.

Third, many adult children become so far drawn into their parents' problems that their own lives suffer. Time and energy they spend dealing with or worrying about their parents can compromise participation in their own family and marital relationships.

Finally, the triangulation process no doubt interferes with rehabilitation from illness, regardless of where on the triangle the heart patient is positioned. A heart patient who is overaligned with a grown child to the exclusion of his or her spouse will suffer the pain of lessened marital intimacy. If the heart patient is the excluded member of the triangle, rehabilitation will be complicated by the difficult emotions of loneliness and isolation that come with this position. And if the heart patient is in the role of negotiator of unresolved conflict between two other family members, then that patient's already compromised physical functioning will be further hurt by the stress of being caught in a family triangle.

Adding complexity to this picture is the fact that triangles are not always confined to the mother-father-child triad. Particularly for adult children in family systems, the invitations to triangulate can come from several generations. This situation can become quite complex as a sheer function of numbers. For example, in a family of two children, two parents, and four grandparents, the number of family triangles simultaneously available to any one person is twenty-one. And this number does not even take into consideration the possibility that the grown children in this family may have children of their own.

The story of the Thibodeaux family demonstrates how complex family triangulation can become in the lives of adult children of heart patients.

Renée Thibodeaux and her husband, Adam, were settling into a stage of comfortable security after eighteen years of marriage. Three years before, they had moved to a suburb of New Orleans, where their extended families lived. Renée and Adam were happy to be living near their aging parents at last, after having lived all over the Northeast because of Adam's multiple career moves. They were thriving: Adam was enjoying being in the prime of his career, Renée was rapidly climbing the ranks in her own work as a real estate broker, and their three teenage children were flourishing in their school and extracurricular involvements.

Then Renée's mother had a massive heart attack, and everyone's life began to change. Adam and the children were very supportive of Renée's increased involvement with her parents at first. They assured her of their blessings as she absented herself from them to help her frightened parents adjust to this unexpected crisis.

With Renée's help, her parents adjusted quite nicely. After three months of closely monitoring and participating in their lives, Renée began to skip calling on her parents for a few days at a time and to focus her energies once again on her own family and her career. Her parents, of course, had been encouraging Renée to trust that they would be all right and to spend time with her husband and children. They were concerned for their grandchildren and for their son-in-law as well as for themselves.

All was going as well as could be expected by the sixth month of Grandmother's rehabilitation when a subtle shift in the family patterns occurred. Renée's father began to drop hints to Renée that her mother was spending long periods of time crying, refusing to get out of bed, and lamenting her poor health. Grandmother was depressed. In his talks with Renée, Grandfather became progressively more open in his expressions of concern for his wife. The two of them developed multiple strategies for encouraging and facilitating Grandmother's return to a more full and active involvement in her life.

Daily phone conversations with her parents and frequent visits once again became Renée's predominant focus. She had many private conversations with her father to get "progress reports" on her mother. She tried to act cheerful and encouraging when dealing directly with her mother, but the concern that she shared only with her father began to feel like a family secret that was placing a strange feeling of distance between Renée and her mother.

Renée's stress level mounted as tension began to develop between herself and her only sibling, Loretta, who began to question Renée's handling of their parents' efforts to recover. Loretta lived in another state and, through periodic phone calls and letters, noticed her mother's growing depression; she encouraged Renée to "visit Mama and Daddy more often." In response, Renée felt understandably angry and unappreciated. Here she was, changing her life out of concern for her parents, and her sister was accusing her of not caring enough to visit more often!

Further fueling Renée's anger was the tension that was mounting between herself and her husband. Adam began to complain about her increased absences during evenings and weekends, reminding her that he and their children needed and missed her. Renée, too, was frightened and distressed by the eroding intimacy in her own family. Even when she was home, she was often upset and preoccupied with her mother's health and with her father's worries and fears. Three generations of her family were in a shambles, and her own career was suffering.

As tension between Renée and Adam led to a cool distancing within the marriage, Renée's second child, Robert, began to serve as her confidant and nurturer. This son, who had always been the emotionally sensitive peacemaker in the family, was an inevitable participant in the family drama. Robert began to express concern to Renée that she was worrying herself into exhaustion. He encouraged her to take a break from nursing her parents, offering to spend weekends with them himself so Renée could travel with Adam or just relax or catch up on her mounting backlog of work. He also began to bicker with Adam, accusing him of not understanding the pressures that faced Renée. In gradual and subtle ways, Robert began to organize his life around his concerns about his mother and his parents' relationship. Soon the son was as extensively involved in the drama between Renée and Adam as Renée was involved in her own parents' adjustment difficulties.

In the nine months following Grandma's heart attack, the Thibodeaux family had become filled with tension and with triangular patterns of struggle. Renée was caught in a triangle with her parents and in a similar pattern involving her husband and her son. Robert was triangulated between Renée and Adam. And Adam, feeling left out of everything, was at high risk of triangulating either another of the Thibodeaux children or one of his own extended kinfolk as his ally against the growing tension. Finally, tension between Renée and her sister, Loretta, was growing, thereby increasing the likelihood that yet another family triangle would develop.

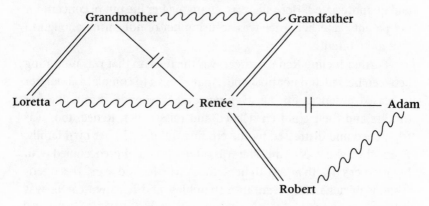

Unless properly handled, such family processes have a negative effect on the physical, marital, and family health of all parties involved. But what is to be done in this situation? After all, no self-respecting person feels good about turning his or her back on ailing loved ones during their times of need. And no loving parents want any of their children to get caught in a stress-filled trap.

Avoiding family closeness is certainly not the solution to family triangulation. Rather, the task is to recognize and change patterns of triangulation while increasing efforts to relate more healthily to the other family members. Doing so may require behavior changes on the part of both the parents and the children.

What Parents Can Do to Help

To begin with, parents should learn to be aware of signs that they may be turning to their children for support in unhealthy ways. If you are having marital problems that you are not facing together, then the risk increases that your children will become unhealthily involved in the family drama. Any number of marital patterns or problems can increase the odds of triangulation occurring within the family:

- Excessive emotional dependency of the medical patient on the spouse.
- Indirect communication style within the marriage.
- The couple's narrow range of social contacts, paired with excessive emotional dependency on the children.
- Difficulty in resolving marital conflict.
- Sexual problems between the spouses.
- Generally poor intimacy between the spouses, perhaps due to difficulty in directly expressing warmth and affection.
- Spouses feeling misunderstood by or disinterested in each other.

Of course, this list is far from complete. Also, a couple can evidence all the foregoing problems and still not triangulate their children. But the point is that *if you are having marital problems, the tensions between you increase the odds that one or more of your children will become involved in the drama.*

While you are honestly examining the status of your marriage and family patterns, it helps to be sensitive to signs that any of your children are behaving in ways that create communication triangles. You may not intend for your children to become involved in your problems; these grown-up children with minds of their own may simply be barging into your private life uninvited. Regardless of why they are doing so, the important point is for you, as loving parents, to try to keep your children from assuming responsibility for your emotional life.

For example, invitations to one parent to gossip about the other, however lovingly phrased, usually signal that the child is responding to tensions that need to be addressed between husband and wife, not between parent and child. Or such conversations may be a concerned child's way of asking for reassurance that the two of you are taking care of your emotional business. Respond appreciatively to such invitations, but clearly refuse to participate in a negative drama involving one of your children and your spouse. This form of mature response is one of the greatest psychological gifts a parent can give a child of any age. Giving children unnecessarily private information about your marriage is harmful, both to your marriage and to your child. To do so is to weave one of the worst psychological webs that trap children and strangle their growth as individuals.

How should you respond, then, if a child expresses concern for your marriage? First, here is an example of a poor response: "Thank God you asked! I've been going out of my mind worrying about your daddy. He's just not the same since his heart attack, and he and I just aren't getting along. I don't know what to do! Maybe if you talked to him it would help. He does seem to brighten up when you and the kids come to visit. Maybe you should come over more often."

By responding this way, you would convey to your child the message, "You should feel responsible for solving this problem that exists between your parents." Such pressure will only increase your child's distress level.

A far more healthy and caring response to your child's expression of concern for your mate might be: "I appreciate you and your concern. Your dad is having some struggles right now that are sometimes hard to understand and to live with. But we are dealing with them. Being married teaches you how to get through hard times, and this is a hard time that we'll lick one way or another. We both love you and know you love us, and that's important to us. But this is something that he and I have to deal with."

The point is not to shut your concerned children out of your emotional life. The point is to reassure them that they are free to live their own lives, and that with love, support and caring, you will deal with your own marital struggles.

If you and your spouse realize that you are triangulating one of your children, then simply stop! Read this book together and speak to each other about your own struggles with intimacy or the fears that are keeping you from settling your marital issues. Then, with a sense of "we-ness," speak with your loving children, and free them from their sense of responsibility for your emotional well-being.

It may be particularly soothing to your child to learn that you have employed someone else, such as a professional marital therapist, to help you. This freeing of your child from triangulation can be done with laughter and should be done with open statements of appreciation and love for each other. For example:

"We appreciate your coming over to talk with us. We want you to know about some new developments with us. We've been learning some things about how families work, and we realize that we had you caught in the middle of our tensions. This isn't a good place for you to be, and we're learning that this pattern in families just keeps marriages stuck in these issues.

So we wanted to let you know that we're firing you as our marriage therapist. Your replacement is going to be Dr. _____. You have two weeks to move your counseling operation to another troubled marriage. We love you, but you can't work for us any longer."

Impossible as it may seem to imagine having such a conversation with your children, I assure you that such words would be music to the ears of any child caught in parents' relationship tensions. We harbor hopes and fantasies that our loved ones will be well and will care lovingly for each other. One of the many hard tasks of parenting is freeing children from their concern and their sense of responsibility for their parents' relationship.

What Adult Children Can Do to Help

The family meeting just described may seem awkward to pull off, but a much more difficult and emotionally painful feat faces adult children who must free themselves from a parental triangle *without* the blessing or cooperation of the parents. Most people caught in their own versions of the Thibodeaux family struggle ultimately face a painful decision: they must choose to control their degree of participation in their family's various dramas, because the dramas will continue forever.

In her excellent book, *The Dance of Anger,* Harriet Goldhor Lerner points out that family members caught in triangles must learn to get out of the middle of tension between loved ones. Furthermore, she recommends the practice of preventive medicine: learn to avoid getting triangulated in the first place, and your family life will go more smoothly.[2]

Even when other family members are not appropriately managing their own lives or their relationships with each other, you are well advised to learn to create, tolerate, and maintain an appropriate degree of involvement with them. Here are eight helpful suggestions for handling complicated family triangles.

1. Stay calm when dealing with conflicting family relationships. Anxiety and an inner sense of urgency are the driving forces underlying triangles.

2. Stay out of the relationships between other family members. Do not advise, analyze, criticize, blame, attempt to fix, or take sides.

3. Instead, casually and caringly express your confidence in the abilities of both of the other parties in the potential triangle to resolve their differences or to survive their lack of resolution: "I know that must be hard for you, and I sure do hope things get better. I love you both, and I hope you'll work this out. You know more about this sort of stuff than I do."

4. Maintain a warm, nonjudgmental, nonreactive position, even if you have to react to persistent invitations to gossip. Here is an example of a caring, yet direct, refusal to be triangulated:
   "You know, Mom, it's uncomfortable for me when you talk about Dad with me that way. I know you're worried, and I do want you to feel better. But I love both of you. Plus, I don't know how to solve your problems. When I come to

[2]H. Lerner, *The Dance of Anger: A Woman's Guide to Changing the Patterns of Intimate Relationships* (New York: Harper & Row, 1985).

visit, I like it best if you and I talk about you and about what's going on in my life. When I'm with Dad, I like to talk about him and about me. I don't like to gossip about either of you to the other. So, why don't we talk about _____."

5. If you are angry with one family member, deal directly with that person. Do not triangulate another family member by complaining to him or her that you are frustrated about being triangulated by others.

6. Do not keep or promote secrets between yourself and another person in your family, particularly if you and that person are in different generations.

7. Be open and honest in communicating with your family, but do so without gossiping or blaming another when reporting information. For example, it is perfectly appropriate to respond to a caring inquiry from a concerned family member with such statements as, "Yes, it's true that Betty and I are trying to figure out a new way to deal with our differences. This is hard to do, and we're both struggling right now."

8. Hang in there! This means two things. First, it is important to not turn your back on family members just because interacting with them is uncomfortable for you. Changing relationship patterns feels awkward until the new way of relating becomes more familiar. No healthy changes in family patterns can occur if you simply distance from each other.

    Second, hanging in means enduring the inner anxiety that you will feel as you begin to relate more healthily to your loved ones. This discomfort does not mean you are doing something wrong or something you should not do. It simply means that in being more honest and healthy in your reactions, you have changed some of the steps in a familiar dance with these family members, and they have not yet learned how to respond.

Learning to control yourself and your own reactions is the crucial key to dealing with family triangles. It is a lesson well worth learning. If you are overinvolved in the problems of others in your family, you are probably making two mistakes: (1) You are diverting energy away from dealing with your own life (your problems, your marriage, your family); and (2) you are helping the family members with whom you are triangulated to stay stuck in their relationship problems.

Get out of there! Leave their relationship alone, and they may just surprise you with their individual and collective abilities to change or begin dealing with their old problems in new and healthier ways. There is only one guarantee: if you stay stuck in a family triangle, you increase the odds that someone in the triangle will become more symptomatic.

Summary

Healthy family reactions—to illness or to simple day-to-day life—require that parents remain the architects of the family. As long as you are able to do so, it is important for you to care for each other appropriately. Your loving connection as mates provides an umbrella of security and psychological structure beneath which your children can grow and thrive. Do not fold that umbrella just because heart illness has entered your life.

Regardless of the ages of your children or of your parents, highly stressful times carry with them the risk that someone will become caught in triangulation patterns. To do so is damaging to your marriage and your health.

If you are a cardiac couple living in the "sandwich" generation—feeling responsibilities to your own spouse and children but also feeling responsible to care for aging parents—be especially careful to stay out of multigenerational emotional triangles. Speak openly and lovingly to your parents about your dilemma and about your need to balance your energies both in your family of origin and in your family by marriage. Accept that you cannot be the perfect son or daughter, even if your parents have difficulty believing it. Be loving. Be available. But be clear that your primary energies must be directed to living your own life.

If you are a cardiac couple with grown children, try to maintain a balance between respecting your children's needs for independence and being open with them about your needs. It is all right to ask for support, help, guidance, or companionship from your children. I hope you have already taught them that it is safe to speak their minds in dealing with you. If they are available and willing to give what you ask, then so be it. But if your children indicate through their words, their actions, or their own symptoms that they are caught in a conflict of loyalties, then give them your blessing to focus their energies on coping with their own problems. You remain the parents and they the children, through all the days of your life together. Free them to live by loving each other.

Finally, let me emphasize that no family fulfills all the glowing descriptions of healthy functioning, and no family is all bad. The descriptions of positive and negative family characteristics in the preceding several chapters are presented in the hope that you may be able to identify yourself and make changes in your life if you need to. Viewing yourselves from the foregoing perspectives can be quite helpful in stimulating growth within your family. I recommend that you use and reuse these chapters as blueprints to guide you during times of discussion in your marriage and in your family relations. Remember that normal, healthy families are those who continue to grow and change together; a steady state of perfection is never attained or maintained in family teams.

If your family is struggling in its efforts to adjust to heart illness, it is likely that either a cause or an effect of this struggling is lessened marital intimacy. The remainder of this book is devoted to what I consider one of the most important aspects of cardiac rehabilitation: marital intimacy.

Part II

· · · · · ·

Intimacy: The Key to Health

Seven

Pictures of a Healthy Marriage

■ ■ ■ ■ ■ ■

It has been said that the patient may recover from his coronary but that his wife may not. She has often seen her husband when he looked near to death, she may have been warned that he could die. . . . She has the same fears, lack of knowledge, and misconceptions as her husband. . . . Months after the infarct many wives report that they lie awake listening to their husbands' breathing to make sure that he is still alive. . . . She may also collapse under the strain of anxiety, become sick, depressed, develop chest pains. . . . Alternatively, wives may take over decision-making and bread-winning roles and become highly overprotective; this may increase the patient's feelings of helplessness and despondency.[3]

I have never met a heart patient's spouse, male or female, who could not relate to this quotation. The secret that haunts many cardiac marriages is the spouse's unexpressed and unsoothed agony over the current and future struggles that this myocardial invasion has brought into the couple's life.

My interest in working in cardiac rehabilitation has endured primarily because of my experiences with the spouses of the cardiac pa-

[3]J. Crawshaw, Community rehabilitation after acute myocardial infarction, *Heart and Lung* 3 (1974):258.

tients whom I have treated. In fact, as a marriage and family specialist, I have spent almost as much time with cardiac spouses as I have with heart patients themselves. What I have learned and continue to learn from these brave and overstressed men and women has been a fascinating set of lessons on how healthy and unhealthy marriages are created and maintained.

The stress of cardiac rehabilitation seems to bring out the best and the worst in marriages. Almost all partners are able to put aside their differences at least momentarily and rekindle mutual affection or further fuel existing love and commitment to each other during the initial scare when illness changes their lives. However, as the case examples presented here illustrate, the many stresses that accompany cardiac rehabilitation inevitably seem to create problems in *sustaining* comfortable intimacy. I propose that the question is not whether your marriage will be affected by heart illness and cardiac rehabilitation; the question is, How are you doing in your efforts to overcome the negative impact that this illness had or is having on your marital relationship?

In the pages that follow, I describe how healthy marriages—those that maintain a reasonably high degree of intimacy and passion—develop and grow. Next, I disclose the secrets of establishing and maintaining intimacy in marriage and discuss the very important topic of sexual functioning and heart illness. And I give special consideration to the ways personality factors, especially those that have to do with Type A personalities, affect marital reactions to illness.

In my clinical practice, I usually begin marital therapy by coaching and educating the couple on the concepts described in the upcoming pages. I invite you to pretend that you are now paying me to sit with you in my cozy office to say out loud to you all the words printed on these pages. If you pretend you have paid a small fortune to hear these recommendations for enhancing your marriage, you are much likelier to follow through on the suggestions I make.

The Stages of Marriage

Falling in love and getting married is easy. Staying married is not all that difficult, either. Even when the marriage is not a happy one, many couples decide just to endure; they decide that they are trapped with each other, and then they live semimiserably ever after.

Keeping your marriage alive and growing, on the other hand, is a most difficult challenge, and it is also no doubt the most rewarding and healthiest of the alternatives that face you once you vow, "I do." Understanding how your marriage developed and where you are now on your path of growth as a couple can be very helpful in this regard.

Just as individuals continue in their psychological growth throughout life, marriages likewise progress through fairly predictable stages of change. Understanding these stages of marriage and their underlying psychological and emotional issues can greatly calm the turmoil that naturally occurs when illness threatens to stop the growth of your relationship. In the following pages, I describe marriage as having three major stages, each of which involves certain dramas or themes that tend to organize much of the emotional reacting and counterreacting that make up day-to-day living as a couple. I emphasize that this is only a theoretical conceptualization of marriage; no marriage actually progresses clearly through each of these steps of growth, and there is no way to predict how long it will take for a given couple to grow from one stage to the next.

Finding the Ideal Mate

Each of us begins life in what might be called our *homestead*, which is our first family experience. Because the world is an imperfect place and none of us is blessed by being the center of the universe, we leave our first family with the wounds and insecurities that result from not being loved perfectly. When we leave the homestead, we take with us a primitive hope that we will find someone who will love and accept us enough to heal our emotional wounds and quiet our insecurities.

Unfortunately, many of our initial attempts to find that perfect connection prove to be false starts. Our own and other people's immaturities produce further hurts and disappointments. This negative drama of searching continues far too long for most of us. We begin to feel as though we are floundering. We are looking for an intimate island of refuge from our insecurities and for a partner with whom to share our life, but we begin to fear that we may never reach our goal.

Finally, however, we fall in love and are loved in return by someone who seems to be our dream come true. The other person seems to fulfill our hope of being loved perfectly. Of course, our image of this other person is influenced to a great degree by our own fears and fantasies. At this stage of our development, we tend to see what we need to see and to be what we need to be in order to create harmony with another person. The alternative—continued floundering alone—is too frightening.

This is an important point: *No matter how healthy a marriage ends up being, it probably started out based on mutual unrealistic hopes about who each person would be in the other's life.* The bliss we experience at the beginning of a relationship results from the excitement that comes from transferring our primitive needs into the belief that we have found the perfect person to satisfy those needs. At this stage, our future spouse may appear to be the answer to our unconscious prayer to find a perfect "parent"—a person who will end our searching and loneliness by making us the center of his or her universe; a person who will love us back so well and so thoroughly that all the wounds and insecurities we have collected in life thus far will soon be erased.

Our choice of mate at this stage leaves us feeling as though we will finally live happily ever after. No small part of our excitement at this point is attached to the hope that in marrying this partner we will be able to finesse growing up. We hope to be able to skip the hard work of self-development simply by marrying someone who possesses the qualities we find lacking in ourselves. We hope to learn to be more outgoing, loving, strong, stable, fun loving, or whatever we are not, simply through affiliation with this new partner. A secondary hope is that we will make a similar difference in our spouse's development: "In me, my future mate has finally found someone who will love away all of life's wounds and all of his or her imperfections."

But then the troubles begin. Behind every mountain is a valley, and sometime after the initial glow of marriage begins to fade, we begin to notice signs of doubt. This second stage is signaled by growing concerns about why our partner's love is not perfectly soothing, as we had expected it to be.

Struggling to Change Each Other

At first, this second stage of marriage involves a growing awareness of the limits to which our own developmental pains will be soothed by this relationship: "No matter how talkative my wife is, I'm still shy." "No matter how laid back my husband acts, I'm still a workaholic." "No matter how much she models social drinking for me, I'm still alcoholic." "No matter how nurturing he acts, I still feel unloved."

Sooner or later this awareness leads us to complain, privately or to someone else, about our partner's failure to change: "I'm nurturing him as much as I can, but he still has a violent temper." "I thought when we got married that she just needed a tender lover to help her to trust men again, but she's still just as cold and distant as ever." "I figured that once we had kids he'd have a reason to take better care of himself, but he just keeps on working himself to death."

As frustrations and fears mount, the marriage enters a stage filled with struggles. The couple struggle to change each other enough to (1) make a positive difference in their individual struggles with their own psychological issues and (2) match their images of who they thought the other person was when they first met. Couples in this stage of marriage use many methods of trying to make each other change to fit their ideal:

They may say, "You promised": "You promised you would stop working such long hours after we got married. Here it is six years later, and you're away from home more than ever."

They may accuse, "You've changed": "Why do you always harp on this? You knew I was serious about my career when we got married, and you didn't say a word about it then. You knew what you were getting when you got me. I'm just being me; *you've* changed."

They may plead, "For the sake of": "For the sake of our children, if not for me, please learn to control your temper." "For the sake of your own health, you have to learn to slow down and not worry so much." "For God's sake, why don't you start enjoying life like you used to when we first met?"

The struggle heats up as neither person gives in to the other's requests for change. As they realize that they will not achieve change through any of these methods, a couple may try a new tactic. One spouse may assume the role of the pursuer, always seeking information, communication, contact, and intimacy from the other. The other spouse becomes the distancer, always reacting with distraction, fatigue, disinterest, worry, absence, or some other form of avoidance of intimacy.

The more the first person pursues, the more the second person distances, and the more the first person pursues. Finally the pursuer gets fed up or fatigued and starts to withdraw or give up, only to find that the distancer is suddenly interested in connection. Delighted with this turn of events, the pursuer becomes available, but the distancer then backs off, and the pursuer-distancer dance continues. Observing such couples reminds me of watching two magnets of the same charge chase each other about a table, never able to come into direct contact.

As frustration in this stage of marriage grows, the couple begins to lament, silently or aloud, the way the marriage has turned out. A growing awareness develops: "This is no dress rehearsal; this is the only life I've got to live, and I'm tired of this struggle." Things really heat up as one partner's struggle to get the other to change drifts into accusations such as, "The older you get, the more you remind me of your mama [or daddy]." (This is a surefire way to elicit irrational anger from your spouse during an argument. Don't try it!) When these accusations also fail to create miraculous changes in the marital process, partners begin to lament their lot in life: "I'm afraid we might have gotten married for more wrong reasons than right reasons."

Truly Accepting Each Other

Whenever a couple voices to me the fear that they may have married for more wrong reasons than right reasons, my reply is, "Of course you did. Most of us did. What did we know about the realities of marriage when we started out? The fact that you had a bunch of vague, rather unrealistic hopes about each other and about what marriage would be does not mean you made a mistake, or that you have a bad marriage. What happens *next* will determine whether you have a good marriage."

For healthy couples, what happens next is called *differentiation*. They begin to grapple with the awareness that the marriage can soothe pains or fulfill needs only to a certain extent. They become aware that we all have certain feelings of aloneness or emptiness that cannot be soothed by our mates, no matter how healthy the marriage becomes.

Further, they become truly aware of the limits on how much each of us is capable of changing another person. For cardiac couples, this is a particularly painful point. They need to confront openly the fact that the spouse cannot rehabilitate the heart patient. No matter how much loving, preaching, role modeling, or reading the spouse does, it is up to the heart patient to decide whether to adjust to the illness in healthy ways. This awareness often leaves both partners feeling alone as they struggle with the truth—that the marriage can help, but it cannot heal all their individual wounds and worries.

Once the couple has differentiated in this way, the challenge becomes one of understanding the emptiness felt within. They must learn to distinguish between emptiness that is caused by the other spouse and emptiness that is simply part of being human and being aware of the accumulated pains of life. The challenge at this juncture is to block the tendency to run from this pain. Some people try to numb themselves with drugs or food. Others try to distract themselves from their pain by pursuing other relationships or compulsions. Neither of these responses results in further growth or satisfaction.

Enduring this pain rather than running from it takes couples through a stage of despair when each of them becomes truly aware of the limits on what will come from the marriage. Fortunately, this stage, the stage of marital growing pain, is often relatively brief. Partners who do not run from each other begin rather quickly to develop a new, more mature, and less dream-come-true understanding of the goodness of their marriage. Unhealthy couples tend to disintegrate at this point, refusing to accept that no marriage can perfectly soothe both partner's pains all the time. Healthy couples begin to mature by psychologically differentiating; they become more accepting of their individual differences, and they begin to calm the power struggles that by now have grown tiresome and frightening for both of them. A new kind of peace and loving acceptance of each other begins to develop.

In this period of growth, each partner continues the process of differentiation by becoming more familiar with himself or herself. Each becomes more honest and realistic in identifying his or her own underlying emotional needs. And each begins to find more effective and healthy ways to request and accept soothing responses from his or her mate.

These new ways of perceiving oneself lead each partner to form new impressions of the other. The couple then enters a smoother stage in the marriage, in which each partner begins to truly understand the emotional wounds that the other brought into the marriage and begins to understand both the limits and the power of the marriage to heal these wounds. Moments of defensiveness and anger are more lovingly resolved as each spouse learns to respond with increased gentleness to signs that the other is feeling afraid or vulnerable. In addition, when their internal anxieties are not adequately soothed by their partners, they now begin to implement appropriate self-nurturing strategies rather than pout and wallow in pain. Rather than stay stuck in the conscious or unconscious modes of self-centeredness that characterized many of the previous stages of the marriage, they now begin to view each other in more calming and loving ways. They begin to discover or rediscover the endearing aspects of each other's personalities and of their partnership.

Each partner now begins to appreciate the other in new ways. A renewed appreciation blossoms. But now this loving impression of the other is not viewed through the rose-colored glasses of immature and unrealistic expectations about love and marriage. Rather, couples consciously begin to examine the basic questions that underlie marriage: Do we accept the limits on how much our marriage can soothe our internal psychological struggling? Do we still choose to face the challenge of living as two separate people who work lovingly to be healing partners in this complicated but worthwhile experience of being married?

For couples who choose to continue the journey, marriage now becomes a quest to learn how to relate in ways that are healing for each other. In so doing, they begin the final stage of the marital journey by entering what might be called *Good Enough Territory*. Each partner in a thriving couple settles into this territory of Good Enough, accepting the other's lack of perfection and focusing energies on being as good a mate and as nurturing a partner as possible.

The Secret of Intimacy

My wife, Mary, is my partner in professional practice. Since the late 1970s, we have noticed that the couples we treat tend to fall into two broad categories. On the one hand are people who lament that the flame is gone from their relationship. They often seem demoralized and discouraged about the possibility of maintaining passion in marriage. On the other hand are the couples who give us hope for our own future and renew our faith and belief in the goodness of marriage. These are the couples who show mutual respect, love, and passion for each other. They describe their marriage as being their "saving grace" or their "constant island of refuge" in life. You can spot them in a minute: they laugh freely, compliment each other openly, and hold hands in our waiting room.

What makes the difference between these two types of marriages? Mary and I have asked ourselves this question for twelve years while observing thousands of marriages. The answer isn't what you would expect. The difference isn't based on educational level, socioeconomic status, size of family, or age. Young or old, rich or poor, childless or living with a house filled with toys and diapers—none of these factors determines whether the couple maintains intimacy as they progress in their marriage.

No, the difference is that successfully married couples know the secret of an intimate relationship. For a relationship to *work*, you need *communication*. But you need to balance problem-solving with *fun* and *cherishing*. *Trust* is essential, and it is created with *fairness* and *commitment*. By giving each other *permission to be complete persons* and by *forgiving* yourselves and each other for your imperfections, you can remain in love as you create a life together. Now, a few thoughts about each of these factors.

Work

Healthy couples accept that relationships don't work unless we work on them. This basic belief is quite contrary to the myth of naturalism that underlies dysfunctional relationships, which goes something like this: "If we are married [or if we share an office, or if we are neighbors, or if we are in any sort of relationship], then we are supposed to get along naturally. If we don't get along naturally, then something is wrong with one of us, and it probably isn't me!"

The truth, of course, is that no relationship works out naturally. Few things in life are as complicated as an intimate relationship. As we grow and change, what we need and want from intimate others also changes. Maintaining intimacy in a long-term relationship therefore involves constantly relating, as is implied by the term *relationship*. This means that any relationship involves a significant amount of effort. To negotiate the endless series of compromises, hurdles, and developmental passages that are encountered as we live together, couples must *work on the relationship*.

Healthy couples accept this need for work as a fact of being married. Unhealthy couples lament when they encounter some rocky stretch in their relationship, complaining and fearing that this need to work at getting along means their relationship is in trouble. Healthy couples respond to rocky times as proof that they are progressing down the path of growth as a couple, and they understand that this path always contains some stretches of rough going.

When faced with times of significant stress in your marriage, remember that neither of you planned for this to happen. Let yourselves join together and accept that such periods of struggle affect both of you and require you to do extra work as a couple. Getting through such periods is easier if you keep in mind that some degree of work is an inevitable part of any journey that is worth taking. Join in a team effort to overcome the hurdles that face you, and you will continue on the path of relationship growth.

Communication

Much of the work in healthy marriages involves communicating. Intimacy can grow in a relationship only if both people are able to do a reasonable job of accurately identifying and clearly expressing inner thoughts, feelings, needs, and wants. Intimate partners relate to each other in certain ways that promote effective communication. There are no special tricks; good communicators are basically attentive and responsive listeners.

In dealing with each other, your communication will improve if you follow these guidelines:

Closely examine your impressions instead of trying to read minds. Do not assume that your impressions are valid. Get confirmation from the other person.

Speak in *I* language. Use such phrases as "I feel _____," "In my opinion _____," and "I'm afraid that _____."

Avoid statements that blame or shame the other person, even if the statements are phrased in *I* language. Don't say things like, "I feel that you are the reason why our children never come to visit us."

Stick to the topic when attempting to resolve conflict. Don't scatter your focus, and don't bring up old battles as a way of trying to win a current one.

Create communicative environments as the first step in solving important problems. For example, schedule a time to talk in private, and eliminate distractions such as the television, other people in the room, and phone calls.

Develop communication-promoting rituals that are part of daily or weekly life. Specify these as times to touch base with each other. Such rituals might include sitting in the den for thirty minutes before dinner each day and talking, taking walks together, or going out to breakfast together on Saturday mornings.

Look at each other while talking.

Indicate concern for and understanding of each other during conversations by making reflective statements—statements that let the other person know you are hearing what he or she is saying.

Acknowledge your own difficulty in responding reasonably if attempts to resolve conflict are getting nowhere, and suggest a time out from further discussions until you can give a more reasonable response.

Sandwich points of negative feedback between points of positive feedback.

Always apologize to each other following times of conflict. This is not the same as admitting fault; it simply involves saying to the person you love, "I'm sorry we argued. I don't like it when things are tense between us."

This list is, of course, incomplete. However, it provides a starting point for communication. Here are some additional aspects of communication to keep in mind:

Intimate partners communicate in ways that make interacting with each other feel safe and rewarding.

Being open with another person involves being vulnerable to that person. Remember this not only when you're communicating to someone but also when someone is communicating openly with you, and respond appropriately.

We continue being open about our inner feelings, thoughts, needs, and wants only with people who are gentle, caring, and affirming in response to our openness.

All partners make mistakes occasionally in responding to each other. Getting it right the first time around is not very important. Getting it straight after you've gotten it wrong is, however, of utmost importance. To do so, you must communicate effectively.

Fun

Intimate couples regularly have fun together. They laugh frequently. They are playful and sometimes silly in their private ways of relating to each other. They continue to make playing together a priority in their lives, even as additional important responsibilities get added to their "to do" lists.

Unhealthy couples stagnate from working all the time—at jobs, on their house, on their children, or even on their relationship. Speaking of this point, the father of a colleague of mine once remarked: "There is a danger in spending too much time examining a relationship; talking about it, checking it out, constantly processing its workings. It's sort of like taking care of a valued plant—not just by watering it, feeding it, and pruning it—but by constantly pulling it up to look at the roots to see if they are still okay."

Mary and I believe the single most frequent factor that separates intimate couples from stale ones is whether the partners have regular dates with each other. Alive couples regularly treat each other to interludes of fun and entertainment. They make plans in advance to fill such times with interesting activities or conversation. They save their energies and use their resources to participate in such times with enthusiasm and charm, just as they did when they first met and began dating. No wonder they stay in love! They use their "good stuff" to be pleasant and pleasing to each other.

No matter how complex life gets or how limited in extra time or money they are, these couples continue to make space in their lives for regularly experiencing special times. These special times might be as simple as a regular Tuesday night date, an occasional long weekday lunch, or, periodically, more elaborate affairs.

One passionate couple with whom I work swears that the secret to their twenty-eight-year-long positive connection has been their willingness to continue to intrigue and romance each other with creative surprises. For example, one of them will occasionally "kidnap" the other, driving to a nearby hotel for a twenty-four-hour escape from life instead of to the supposed destination of their regular evening out. Or one of them will mail the other a written invitation to "an evening of pleasure." The invitation specifies the date, the time, and the dress. All arrangements for the evening, including baby-sitting, are made by the gift giver.

The particulars of what you do on such occasions matter little to most couples. It can be a fancy affair or a simple date to drive around and spend time alone. What does matter is the process of caringly attending to each other.

As a bonus, in the process of orchestrating surprises for your spouse, you'll probably find yourself thinking of other ways to generate intimacy. For example, you'll start paying attention to what your partner says about what he or she is interested in these days, trying something out of the ordinary routine of your life just for the fun of it, and clearly going out of your way to create pleasurable experiences for your partner.

Putting this sort of energy into your marriage ensures that you will not become bored or boring as the years pass. Fun is the fuel of passion in a marriage. If passion is dwindling in your relationship, then it pays to assume that you have become slack in your efforts to create moments and hours of the sorts of experiences that led to your falling in love with each other in the first place. We remain romantically in love with those who romance us. You know what makes your partner smile; use that knowledge to keep the fires glowing in your marriage.

Cherishing

Through all their years together, intimate partners continue to pay each other the special compliments that are regularly paid during the courtship phase of a relationship: they laugh at each other's jokes; they say nice things to each other; each points out what the other does that is right and appreciated; they say nice things about each other to friends and relatives. In short, intimate partners promote positive self-esteem in each other. These people openly value and admire each other.

I often give my patients the following list of positive comments as a reminder to be actively nurturing in their interactions. Although this list looks like a parents' guideline for reacting to children, it is a very effective list to use with each other. Intimate partners seem to understand that our emotional selves operate in the simple ways of children. Consequently, we cannot help responding positively to comments such as these:

"I'm so proud of you!"

"I was bragging about you to someone today."

"It's amazing to me that you're so good at _____" (fill in the blank with one or more talents).

"You're a lot better at _____ than I am. I admire you for that."

"You're one of my favorite people."

"I love to snuggle with you."

"I love you."

"You're amazing! They ought to write a story about you and publish it in the newspaper."

"I was thinking today about all the things that you mean to this family. I really do appreciate you."

"You're a real good _____ (wife, husband, son, daughter, grandchild, grandparent)."

"I'm really proud and happy that you're mine."

"I'm proud to be your wife (husband)."

"You've made a positive difference in my life."

As corny as these phrases may appear on the written page, positive comments like these can be a glue that joins you and your partner emotionally. Such messages help each of you feel safe in remaining open and loving within the privacy of your marriage.

Trust

Intimacy and trust have a circular relationship in marriages: we most trust those with whom we have intimacy, and we develop intimacy only with people we trust.

Contrary to popular notions, I find that trust is typically neither gained nor lost in marriages through single events. Some events, such as extramarital affairs, certainly do take a tremendous toll on the trust factor in a marriage. However, trust is more often maintained or eroded in marriage by less dramatic, day-to-day patterns of interaction than by dramatic or traumatic events.

For intimate partners, trust is the by-product of the workings of the marriage. They avoid the trust-thwarting trap of acting as though their relationship is a power struggle over who is right and who is wrong. Rather, intimate partners act as though each of them has thoughts, impressions, and preferences that make sense, even if their opinions differ. These people validate each other. In so doing, they begin to trust each other. Put another way, we trust people who show that they can see the world through our eyes even though the world looks different from their own perspective.

For example, a trust-generating response would be: "I know it must seem to you that I don't care as much as I used to. As much as I've been worrying about my health, I haven't paid much attention to you. Your feelings make sense in reaction to my behaviors, but my behaviors are giving a false message. I do still love you, I just haven't been showing that love to you as much as I should and as much as I want to."

On the other hand, a trust-squelching response might be: "What are you talking about? Of course I still care about you. You're just feeling insecure and imagining things. You act paranoid every month right before your period starts. Don't take it out on me."

Your partner's perceptions will surely contain at least a few kernels of truth, if not a bushel basketful. To maintain trust, validate the accurate aspects of your partner's impressions. Then share other information needed for your partner truly to understand your perspective.

Fairness

Intimate partners are fair in their dealings with each other. They create a life that does not overwhelm either of them in proportion to what the other is willing to do. I do not mean that intimate relationships always follow a fifty-fifty split of tasks or obligations. Few marital tasks are traded off on a fifty-fifty basis in most households. For example, in most marriages, one person nearly always cuts the grass while another person nearly always cooks the meals. The division of labor is fairly constant for most couples.

The fairness in intimate marriages has to do with each partner being valued for his or her contribution to the relationship. No one person's contributions are considered more important to the overall workings of the marriage than the other's. Correspondingly, intimate partners do not treat one partner's stress, thoughts, or preferences as more important than the other's.

This spirit of fairness is obvious in intimate marriages in many different ways. For example, a husband may depend on his wife to be the family nurturer. In an intimate marriage, this husband does not believe that his career stress is more important or painful than the stress caused to his wife by endless shopping, cooking, chauffeuring, and remembering everyone's birthdays. The wife in this marriage, on the other hand, does not discount the importance of her husband's contributions to their life together. She values him as an active member of the family team, even though his work schedule may make him relatively unavailable for the shopping, cooking, and chauffeuring that fills daily family living.

Intimate partners set up areas of responsibility and then express appreciation to each other for their teamwork. They do not blame each other when they feel overwhelmed with responsibilities and stress. Intimate partners seem to understand that a given day's stress is not necessarily due to some lack of effort or cooperation on the part of the spouse. In marriage and family living, there is more than 200 percent of "stuff" to do in any given time period. Therefore, some tasks always remain undone, even if both partners exert 100 percent effort all the time. Intimate partners are fair and gracious about appreciating each other's efforts toward managing their complex life.

Commitment

For many couples, the level of intimacy dwindles as the marriage goes on. I think this is unfortunate and unnecessary. Such lessening of intimacy will, however, certainly occur if you make the mistake of many couples, who allow the growing number of stressors in their lives to dictate where on the totem pole of priorities they position the important factor of attending to their marriage. As any happily married person knows, this is a mistake. As your years together advance, more and more important areas of responsibility get added to your list of priorities. The list never stops growing: children, mortgages, careers, grandchildren, health concerns, and so on.

If you attend to your marriage only when life allows you time to do so, you will spend less and less time doing so as life goes on. Intimate partners have the same lengthy lists of important areas of responsibility as bored partners, but they continue to place their marriage at or near the top of their list.

Both professionally and personally, I have found that we progress more healthily through life if our needs for intimacy are reasonably well met. We do better in life if we are living in an intimate marriage. Further, it appears that marriages work to the degree that they receive commitment from both parties. The problem that underlies many unsatisfying relationships is lack of commitment to the marriage. Marriage and family life work best if you clearly declare your loyalty to your mate above all other relationships or involvements in your life.

Yes, I mean that you must choose your partner over all else in your life if your marriage is to fulfill its potential. I believe that doing so does not take away from your healthy and loving participation in other meaningful aspects of life. Rather, living in a committed marriage energizes you to be an even more positive parent, friend, worker, relative, church member, recovering heart patient—whatever else is important in your life.

"What a lot of work! I'm not sure this marital intimacy business is worth it," you may say. This is a legitimate point. It is much easier to have a half-baked, lukewarm, functional, but not very intimate marriage than it is to create and maintain an intimate relationship. Indeed, in my opinion nonintimate marriages are the statistical norm; most people settle for functionality and give up the hope and quest for intimacy in their relationships. The reason? Most people are too lazy to commit themselves to the work involved in maintaining intimacy as marriage progresses.

The question of whether the work involved in committing to marital intimacy is worth it to you is, perhaps, comparable to the question of whether the work involved in owning a house versus renting an apartment is worth the payoff. Owning your own home certainly does involve more work; you must compromise endlessly on decisions about spending your time and money on a house. However, the rewards of home owning do seem worth the extra efforts for most of us.

Marital intimacy, too, is certainly a matter of personal choice. However, be clear and honest with yourself about the available options in the quality of your marriage. In this age of "lite" everything— lite beer, lite ice cream, lite crackers—we somehow are getting lulled into pretending that there is an option to have a "lite intimate marriage." Where marriage is concerned, either you heavily commit yourselves and thereby generate intimacy, or you get lite marriage minus the intimacy. You choose. But remember: lite marriage tastes like spaghetti with no sauce, cereal with no milk, a bagel with no cream cheese. . . .

Permission to Be Complete Persons

Getting married does not mean you will stop growing. This fact seems to escape many spouses. In taking the scary step of falling in love and creating a marriage, we all tend to lock in perspectives on each other. We assign and assume roles in the relationship that allow us to fit together comfortably. We eventually outgrow, or grow tired of, these roles. Then the marriage faces the stress of having to reorganize in reaction to our individual changes. Let me elaborate.

In joining together, we tend to see what we need to see in our partner and be what we need to be in order to create harmony in the partnership. In so doing, each of us is creating and participating in a relationship that excludes some important parts of our total self. For example, a strong woman may put aside her own need to be nurtured so that she can fulfill the role of caretaker in the marriage. At the same time, her compliant husband may put aside his own capacity for independent functioning to fit with this partner who has a need to take care of others. He assumes a dependent role in reaction to her assuming a caretaker role.

As life progresses, we all experience an increasing psychological need to express all aspects of our total sense of self. Anxiety-generating events such as illness tend to heighten this need. Particularly as we are faced with aging and its effect on our health, we feel compelled to incorporate into our marriage those aspects of self that we originally put on the shelf when we connected with this particular mate. This means that as we progress in marriage, we experience increasing need to change, both individually and in how we relate to each other. The meek become more outspoken. The angry become more gentle. The fearful become more brave. The seemingly fearless become more aware of insecurities. The compliant become more aware of their own needs.

These changes are first expressed in marriage because marriage is supposed to be the safest place to be psychologically vulnerable and free. Unfortunately, as we have seen throughout this book, any change on the part of one person in a relationship can cause anxiety throughout the relationship. In reaction to such stress, many spouses fail to nurture each other as they grapple with the marital changes that are forced by such individual growth. Nurturing understanding and encouraging such psychological change are hallmarks of an intimate marriage. Healthy partners do not resent each other's growth, even though growth on the part of one partner has real consequences for both.

Unhealthy partners, on the other hand, act as though they are being double-crossed if their partners change in any way. They act as though they had established an ironclad contract to remain the people they were when they married, and they fight any change in this contract.

Unhealthy attempts to prevent a spouse's growth can take many forms. In response to his wife's complaints and concerns about his regular weekend golf tournaments, one man moaned, "I feel double-crossed that she's changed so drastically. She knew I golfed when we got married, and it seemed acceptable to her then. So why not now?" For other couples the intimacy-eroding response may be to tease, make light of, or refuse to participate in some new and important aspect of a mate's life. Leo and Betty provide an example of this mistake.

Betty was an athletic fifty-seven-year-old who had recently returned to part-time pursuit of her college degree. She had also become much more health conscious since the recent death of her father from a stroke. Accordingly, she joined an aerobic dance class, began cooking healthier meals, and significantly tapered her use of alcohol.

Her husband, Leo, however, was a beer-drinking television addict who hated exercise. He constantly complained to Betty about "wasting time acting like some kind of yuppie with all this school and healthiness business." He refused Betty's repeated invitations to join her in exercising or in attending special lectures on topics being covered in her classes.

These two originally came to me for help with their failing sexual relationship. That Betty and Leo were experiencing intimacy difficulties was certainly no surprise. They simply had failed to grow together because of Leo's refusal to participate graciously in Betty's becoming a more complete person. When such emotional stinginess occurs in a relationship, imbalance always follows, and intimacy is compromised.

To grow as a couple, you must keep up with each other's growth. You must make it your business to remain interested in who your partner is becoming and to learn to relate to this new version of your mate. Doing so can lead to continued excitement and intimacy in your marriage.

As important as it is to nurture such growth in each other, it is also important to remember that change always starts from within yourself. No matter how encouraging and nurturing your spouse is about your right to be a complete person, you must give yourself permission to be a complete person if you are to grow. Yes, you chose and agreed to fulfill a certain role during a certain chapter of your marriage or of your individual life, but you are not locked into that role for the remainder of your existence—unless you fail to give yourself permission to change. Intimate couples are made of healthy individuals who grant themselves and each other permission to continue growing throughout all the years of their life.

Forgiveness

Because none of us is perfect, we are certain to make mistakes. As individuals and as couples, we sometimes simply make poor choices. We choose as wisely as we can, sometimes to discover later that a different choice would have been better. We sometimes are mean and unfair to each other. We sometimes behave selfishly with no justification. We sometimes are insensitive to the needs of our partner, and we sometimes are aware of our partner's needs but choose not to respond lovingly.

These "sometimes" occurrences do not make us all lousy individuals and mates. Even the most intimate marriages are often clouded by less than perfect relationship events. But intimate partners do not let such mistakes and painful relationship *events* turn into intimacy-diminishing *processes* in their marriage. They apologize to each other, and they forgive—they forgive each other and they forgive themselves.

Unhealthy relationships, on the other hand, have a cancer called resentment. Resentment results from clinging to anger. Resentment is fueled by blaming. Partners in dying relationships remind me of a seventy-eight-year-old woman I once knew who had fiery black eyes and one motto in life: "Find out who's to blame, and blame that sucker!"

Couples who live in a spirit of forgiveness are able to heal wounds and soothe hurts with relatively little effort. In contrast, it is exhausting and demoralizing to live with someone who does not forgive. I periodically treat couples who change greatly in response to marital therapy but remain miserable. Such people can learn to enhance their communication styles. They can learn to solve problems more fruitfully and to make love more pleasurably. They can learn to understand themselves and each other with more psychological sophistication. They can do all this right stuff, but their efforts do not bear fruit because they do not forgive. Forgiving is like casting away a hot ember that has been placed in your hand. Letting go of this pain frees you to create and to enjoy the balm of continued intimate connection.

Summary

Couples who know the secret of keeping intimacy alive are able to remain in Good Enough Territory and have a reasonably happy and healthy marriage. Such a marriage—what I call "a healing marriage"—is a great aid to coping with the stresses of illness and rehabilitation. In a healing marriage,

1. You accept the challenge of making your relationship a place of nurturing for each other, both in reacting to your partner's childhood wounds and in reacting to your partner's daily stresses.

2. You accept that marriages—like individuals—grow and change, and you never stagnate in your willingness to discover new aspects of each other.

3. You take responsibility for being honest with your partner about what you think, feel, need and want—both on a daily basis and on broad levels regarding what is important to you in your life.

4. You train yourself to behave constructively when relating to your spouse. Rather than getting stuck in destructive ways of communicating, you listen, empathize, and compromise.

5. You privately and publicly convey respect for your partner's thoughts, feelings, needs, and wishes, and you openly let the world know that you value and are proud of your mate.

6. You acknowledge your own negative personality traits, weaknesses, and insecurities, and you work honestly in your efforts to control your defensiveness about them and your tendency to blame your partner for your own struggles.

7. You learn to avoid power-struggle tactics for getting your own needs met, and you replace them with more direct, honest, and fair methods of getting your basic needs and desires satisfied by your mate.

8. You learn to develop within yourself the abilities and traits that you need to feel like a more complete person, rather than relying on your partner to make up your personality deficits for you.

9. You learn to be less driven by stress and frustration, more gentle and forgiving in your dealings with the people in your life, and more balanced in attending to the work and fun aspects of your life.

10. You accept the fact that keeping the spirit of healing alive in your marriage won't happen naturally; it will involve consciously working together to maintain a loving teamwork.

Our discussion of healthy marriages has thus far omitted a crucial ingredient: sex. Many people believe that sexual compatibility is the most important aspect of marital intimacy. This notion is certainly open to debate, but professionals in the field of marital therapy have repeatedly noted that sexual issues are among the concerns most frequently mentioned by couples at all stages of marriage. As will be seen in the following chapter, attending to this very important aspect of marriage is a crucial part of cardiac rehabilitation.

Eight

Sex and Heart Illness

■ ■ ■ ■ ■ ■

One of the many psychological dramas involved in coping with heart disease may surprise you: from the earliest moments following a heart attack, many patients begin worrying about future effects on their sexual abilities. That's right, many people—both men and women—lie on that emergency room bed with a pain in their chest and tears in their eyes and wonder if they will still be able to do "it" like they used to.

Research has suggested that somewhere between 20 percent and 40 percent of heart patients may experience periods of impaired sexual functioning. Research further suggests that an even higher percentage of spouses of heart patients experience anxiety about sex. Many cardiac couples undergo long-term sexual adjustment struggles. Lessened sexual drive for both males and females, impaired ability to get or maintain erections for men, and diminished sexual arousal for women are but a few of the sexual difficulties that can plague couples following heart illness.

But citing data is unnecessary in discussing sexual aspects of cardiac rehabilitation. The fact is that intimacy is our most basic psychological need, and marital intimacy is directly related to sexual intimacy in many ways. Most cardiac patients and their spouses have questions about sex after heart illness. I hope to answer these questions here.

The self-questioning and fears that inevitably come with facing heart disease can seriously erode the many "flavors" of intimacy in your marriage, especially the wonderful flavor of sexual relating. Add to this the fact that much of self-concept is tied to sexuality, and the importance of this topic is obvious.

We are taught from our earliest days to define ourselves as sexual beings. I am not referring to genital sexual experience; I will get to that topic soon. Here, I am referring to our most basic sense of ourselves as being male or female persons. We are taught to value and to evaluate ourselves from this perspective of sexuality. We think of and speak of ourselves and of each other in such terms as, "He's a man's man," or "She's a sexy woman," or "He has those bedroom eyes," or "She has a beautifully feminine figure."

The confusing irony is that, although we are so obviously taught to value ourselves as being sexual, we are taught virtually nothing about how to understand and enhance our sexual functioning. This lack of accurate information about what to expect of ourselves and of each other within the sexual realm is the major cause of the two culprits that typically underlie sexual performance difficulties: performance anxiety and relationship tensions.

I have often counseled couples who have endured years of marital tension and self-doubt because they had mistaken assumptions about what is normal versus abnormal sexual behavior. I have also noticed that sexual miseducation is not necessarily correlated with formal educational level. Many otherwise well-educated people are simply misinformed, or not at all informed, about medical sexual facts.

Our relative ignorance about sex is understandable when you realize that courses in human sexuality were not taught in medical schools until relatively recent years. In fact, extensive education in human sexual functioning is still not part of most medical school curricula. We have all been doing "it" in the dark in more ways than one.

It seems par for the course of rehabilitation that heart patients and their spouses grapple with concerns about their sex life in silence and confusion. Heart patients are notorious for going to their doctors and remaining quiet about their sexual concerns. They then interpret the doctor's silence on this issue as confirmation of their worst fear: that pleasurable lovemaking has to be given up now that heart illness has arrived.

This is simply not the case. Often, doctors are merely unaware of the patients' sexual concerns. Perhaps they do not give the go-ahead because they are not asked. So it is time to get some facts straight. The first important fact to remember is that *heart illness does not have to end full and enjoyable sexual functioning.* More than 80 percent of heart patients are capable of full sexual functioning without any particular physical risks or cardiovascular complications. The other 20 percent of heart patients can also enjoy active sex lives; they may simply need to adjust their lovemaking styles because of physical changes caused by illness, medication, or aging.

The question, of course, is what can be done to continue—or perhaps to create for the first time—a comfortable sexual relationship? The following pages will answer this question.

First, I discuss the problem of differences in levels of sexual drive that plague many couples. Then I outline the various types of sexual dysfunctions that can occur in the normal course of any marriage. Finally, I discuss in detail the critical factors for enjoying your sex life now that you are undergoing cardiac rehabilitation.

Sex Drive

Bear in mind that heart patients and their spouses are not exempt from any of the struggles that affect the sex lives of every other couple. One of these struggles has to do with sex drive; it is a rare couple that is composed of two individuals who have identical sex drives. Differences in levels of sexual energy and interest are normal in marriage. These differences can become heightened during stressful times in a marriage; one member may turn more urgently to sex for soothing of jangled nerves while the other partner is shutting down sexual feelings in response to the effects of stress.

How a couple resolves differences in sex drive has far-reaching effects on the overall quality of the marriage. I have worked with many couples whose marriages have been ruined by their failure to solve this part of the marital puzzle. The person with more sex drive feels controlled by the other's apparent holding back of sexual openness. The person with less sex drive feels coerced and often manipulated by underlying sexual motives on the part of the constantly pursuing partner. The high-drive partner may feel that the other person is less attracted to him or her, and less in love. The low-drive partner may feel valued by the mate only for what he or she can give sexually.

Causes of Sex Drive Differences

Most of us do not accept the fact that people are no different from other species of animals when it comes to variations in sexual energy. The frequency of sexual activity of any group of individuals within every species of animal, including humans, falls into a bell-shaped curve if plotted across a given period of time. In other words, if 100 rabbits are allowed constant access to breedable mates for a given time, and if the number of times each of these rabbits breeds is charted, some average number of breedings will emerge for this group of animals. Some rabbits will breed considerably more frequently than the statistical average; others will breed less frequently. The point is that we do not label the rabbits that breed more frequently as manipulative or nymphomaniac rabbits. We just conclude that those rabbits have more biologically based sexual energy. Similarly, we would not conclude that the rabbits that breed less frequently are angry or holding back or psychologically hung up from their rabbit childhood experiences. We just conclude that those rabbits have less biologically based sex drive.

So it is with human beings. Most people marry people who have biologically based sex drives that differ from their own. And then the trouble starts. The trouble is rooted in the foolish notion that if we love each other enough we will end up being the same. We understand the foolishness of such thinking if we try to apply it to any biological appetite other than sex. After pouting for forty-eight hours, try saying this to your partner with tears in your eyes and exasperation in your voice: "It's just that I figured that after all these years you would *want* to sneeze whenever I want to" (for "sneeze" you can substitute "eat pizza" or "go to the bathroom" or any other biological need).

The truth, of course, is that we are biologically different from each other even if we do love each other. Many psychological, behavioral, and relationship factors can contribute to sex drive struggles between couples, but one physical characteristic that probably has much to do with determining sex drive differences in many couples is the hormone testosterone. Testosterone is typically referred to as the male hormone because it causes the secondary sexual characteristics in men, such as facial hair and deepened voice. However, this hormone is also present in lesser degrees in women.

Testosterone fuels sexual drive in both sexes. Males are especially dependent on testosterone to fuel sex drive, and they require much greater levels of it to maintain their normal levels of sexual desire. This is a somewhat unfortunate fact, because the normal bodily changes that correspond with aging include diminishment of testosterone level, especially in men. Women, too, experience lessening of testosterone levels as they age, and also if they have their ovaries removed during a hysterectomy.

Resolving Sex Drive Differences

One possible solution to sex drive problems is testosterone replacement therapy, which typically involves either injections or oral administrations of testosterone. Although this therapy is considered medically sound and is quite effective for many, it is not a miracle cure. Many individuals do not respond to testosterone replacement therapy with any marked increase in sex drive, and the possible medical complications from the treatment prohibit its usage for many heart patients. High doses of testosterone can cause increased water and salt retention—obvious complicating factors for individuals who suffer from high blood pressure or congestive heart failure.

However, even if your physical differences in levels of sex drive cannot be erased with hormone therapy, there are many ways you can create and maintain an enjoyable sexual relationship. You simply have to work openly and cooperatively together. Couples who live in harmony are generous and accepting of each other's differences. Couples who enjoy their sexual lives are generous and accepting of their sexual differences. They simply tend not to make as big a deal of sex as many other couples do.

The key to managing differences in sex drive is in remaining open, playful, generous, flexible, and appreciative of your partner with reference to this difference. If you do so, you are much likelier to reach some mutually satisfactory compromise. Many couples ruin their sex life by taking it too seriously. They put sex in a special category within their relationship and lace it with magical expectations and ritualized procedures. In this way, they turn their sexual relationship into something that is strained, at best, or downright weird.

For example, many couples relate sexually only according to some fun-inhibiting formula that dictates when, how, and under what circumstances sex may occur. One couple with whom I worked followed this sexual formula: they had sex only if at least seventy-two hours had elapsed since the last time they had had sex; and if they both had had relatively relaxed days; and if they had engaged in considerable amounts of nonsexual physical affection throughout the preceding thirty-six hours; and if they each had at least one glass of wine; and if it was after 9:30 P.M. on an evening before a morning on which neither of them had to arise before 6:30 A.M.; and if the wife waited for the husband to initiate sex play. These two were amazed and appalled once we wrote out the legal-sounding list of *ifs* to which they had attached their right to play sexually. They had become stuck in the habit of acting this way and had never really reexamined whether such carefulness in relating to each other was necessary.

As the years of a marriage go by, most couples narrow the range of situations in which they express sexual affection and the ways they interact sexually. This seems to be a simple function of the fact that in marriage, we develop habitual ways of relating. This relationship pattern becomes a special problem for partners who start off with considerable differences in biologically based sex drive. If you limit the types of situations in which sexual relating is permissible, you will severely limit how frequently you have affectionate sexual encounters. Couples who enjoy their sex life tend to be free and flexible in general when dealing with each other. They openly give and ask for special attention in their marriage.

Notice how the preceding sentence was worded. These people freely ask for and get from each other many special favors in the course of week-to-week living together. They also resist developing rigid patterns of relating to each other. Their favors might include giving back rubs, fetching glasses of water, preparing special meals, and running errands, as well as sexual interactions.

Here are two good rules to follow in being married: (1) Do not be unreasonable or insensitive in what you ask of each other; and (2) do not feel that the other's gift counts only if he or she really, really wants to give it. In other words, you are more likely to remain flexible and generous in your relationship if you do not ask for sexual or behavioral favors that make either of you very uncomfortable. And it is important to view any favor, sexual or otherwise, as acceptable if it is given in a spirit of love and generosity, even though the giver may not be passionately involved in the act of giving.

In this vein, making love or simply giving or receiving sexual pleasure through oral or manual stimulation can be done in a spirit of playful affection. If you get rid of any expectation that both of you have to be sexually aroused, passionately involved, and ultimately orgasmic every time either of you feels sexy, you will greatly relax—and improve—in your sexual relating.

The reason? Such openness and mutual respect lessens tensions that might otherwise accumulate in response to your sex drive differences. By becoming more relaxed about sex, you can avoid becoming tense and emotionally stingy in dealing with each other. This is important, because tension in your relationship can magnify biologically based differences in sex drive. If this happens, you run the risk of accumulating resentments that then erode intimacy throughout your marriage. What begins as a manageable physical difference becomes a seemingly unmanageable fact of life for many couples.

An additional problem for couples caught in this trap is that tensions arising from struggles over sex drive differences can create other problems in sexual performance. As is discussed at length in the following pages, anxiety about sex can cause such problems as impotence and orgasmic dysfunctions.

If you have struggled with frustrations over your sex drive differences, you may first need a period of relationship cleansing and rebuilding before your sexual differences can be addressed. To become playful and generous in the ways described in the preceding paragraphs, you must first come to peace with each other. Only then will you feel safe enough to try new ways of dealing with each other sexually.

Finally, I want to emphasize that it is perfectly normal to experience a lessening of sex drive in conjunction with being physically ill. As we get sick, our bodies experience a shutting down of physical systems in ascending order of importance to our survival. The systems that are least necessary to survival are shut down first, followed by progressively more important ones. The extreme of this process is a coma, in which all but the most primitive of our life-sustaining physical operations are shut down.

Now, sexual relating may be one of the most fun and pleasurable of our needs, but it is also one of our least physically necessary functions. We do not have to have orgasms to survive, so sex drive is very likely to diminish during times of increased physical alarm, such as when coping with illness or with prolonged periods of stress. Be realistic in understanding and accepting this fact, and your sexual energies will return as your body heals.

Sexual Response

The famous sexual researchers William Masters and Virginia Johnson once made the point that every man and every woman periodically experience difficulties in progressing through the sexual response cycle. Every man has periods of erectile failure or of ejaculation control difficulty. Every woman sometimes has difficulty becoming sexually aroused or experiencing climax. This does not mean that we all suffer from sexual dysfunction. It simply means that we all are human and that the human sexual response cycle is rather fickle—contrary to popular mythology, which suggests that all of us "real" men and women are sexual machines, ready to strike as soon as a breedable mate slows down long enough for us to mount.

Sexual dysfunction occurs when a person experiences *persistent* difficulty in progressing through any of the phases of the sexual response cycle.

In understanding your own and your partner's sexuality, it is important to know the basics about the human sexual response cycle. If all goes well during attempted sexual interaction, our bodies progress through fairly predictable stages.

First comes sexual *arousal,* during which time males experience erection because blood is flowing into the penis, and females experience vaginal lubrication and swelling because of similar vascular activity. Next comes the *plateau* phase of arousal. Continued sexual interaction is experienced as pleasurable and results in growing sexual tension and arousal. Finally, sexual tension and arousal culminate in the pleasurable release of *orgasm,* which may or may not be accompanied by ejaculation for males.

Some women are capable of experiencing multiple orgasms, but many women and most men experience a physical *resting phase* following orgasm. During this resting phase (which is sometimes also called the *refractory phase*), the body shuts down the sexual response cycle. Further physical signs of arousal from sexual stimulation may not be possible during this resting phase, even if high levels of mental arousal still exist. In other words, during this sexual resting phase, it may not be possible for a man to gain another erection or for a woman to experience another orgasm, even though they may continue to feel sexy. As one of my patients put it, "After I have an orgasm, I feel so close to my wife and am so attracted to the sight of her body lying next to me that I want to keep making love to her. At that point, I can do all kinds of things in my head, but my penis won't cooperate."

This resting phase begins quite abruptly for men, resulting in rapid loss of erection. A woman's body both turns on and reverses the sexual response much more gradually. I believe that herein lies the reason why many men want to roll over and go to sleep after sex, whereas women tend to want to cuddle, talk, or continue to interact in affectionate or sexual ways. It is not just that we men are insensitive and uncommunicative (even though that may also be true); the abrupt turning off of the sexual response cycle can result in temporary feelings of sleepiness and relaxation.

Although a woman's physical sexual response is more gradually reversed, a woman does not always desire prolonged sexual stimulation. In fact, many women find sexual stimulation unpleasant after orgasm, like the feeling of overstimulation that results if you get tickled for too long.

Another result of this sexual resting phase is diminishment of sex drive. The length of time during which sex drive is quieted after orgasm varies from individual to individual and varies during a person's life. As will be seen in our discussion of the sexual effects of aging, lengthening of the resting phase of sexual response occurs inevitably as we grow older.

Finally, it is important to emphasize that no one always progresses neatly through the phases of sexual response. Rather, you move all along the continuum of sexual responding during a typical lovemaking encounter. You may become highly aroused, then momentarily lose arousal, only to regain it if pleasurable interaction and relaxation continue. In fact, research studies charting penile blood flow during sexual arousal have shown that blood actually flows into and out of a man's penis in a manner that can be charted as an upwardly moving stock market graph. Knowing this fact can help prevent needless anxiety if you notice a momentary lessening of arousal as you are making love. Just relax, and arousal will return.

Sexual Performance Problems

With the matters of sex drive differences and sexual response as a backdrop, let us turn now to discussion of various problems that occasionally interfere with full sexual relating. As you read on, remember that most of us experience each of these forms of sexual problems sometime. The important question is whether you or your partner is experiencing any of these intimacy-squelching sexual patterns consistently.

Arousal Problems

Some people have adequate levels of sex drive but simply have difficulty becoming sexually aroused. Despite high levels of desire, some men find that their penises just will not get erect or stay erect, and some women find that their vaginas just will not become lubricated.

In men this problem is called *impotence,* and it can occur in various forms. Some men cannot attain any degree of erection. Others are able to experience erection but complain that their erections are not hard enough for intercourse. Still other men are able to get erect during foreplay but lose their erections (without experiencing orgasm or ejaculation) before or shortly after beginning intercourse. A special form of impotence that affects a small percentage of men involves being able to ejaculate without an erection. This is possible because erection and ejaculation are controlled by different aspects of the central nervous system.

Finally, some men are able to enjoy full erections throughout the sexual response cycle in certain situations but not during intercourse. For example, some men have no difficulty with erection while masturbating or while receiving manual or oral stimulation from their partner, but they are unable to maintain erection once intercourse begins.

Female sexual arousal difficulties are less evident, for obvious reasons. A man's degree of erection is more easily measured than are the degrees of vaginal lubrication and swelling that signal female arousal. It is therefore more difficult to be exact in describing the variations of arousal problems experienced by women. Let it suffice to say that many women, too, experience high levels of sexual desire but no cooperation from their genitals in response to sexual stimulation. Some such women are able to have reflexive orgasms in response to sexual stimulation, but—like men who ejaculate without erection—they get only limited gratification from this pattern of sexual response.

Orgasm Difficulties

Men can experience two forms of orgasm difficulty: *quick ejaculation* and *retarded ejaculation.* Men who have trouble maintaining control of ejaculation once high levels of sexual arousal are reached have the condition called quick ejaculation. I have worked with countless men who go to dehumanizing lengths to increase their ability to hold off ejaculation. Even though such strategies may allow them to "last longer," quick ejaculation may still happen once the distracting stimulus stops and sexual pleasure is noticed again.

One man I treated developed the habit of abruptly pointing his toes whenever he felt arousal mounting during lovemaking with his wife. In this way, he would cause the insteps of his feet to spasm in pain, thus distracting himself from his pleasurable sexual feelings. He did last a few minutes longer before ejaculating, but his feet surely did hurt after making love. Other men use desensitizing creams or multiple condoms to numb the pleasure of intercourse so as to last a few precious moments more. The problem with these techniques is that they mute all pleasure from sexual relating.

Ruining your sexual pleasure to prolong lovemaking is not a true solution to problems with quick ejaculation. Some men are probably quick ejaculators because of biological factors, but many such men can learn to control ejaculation better if they learn to be *more*, not *less*, aware of and sensitive to their body's progression through the sexual response cycle.

At the opposite end of the spectrum of male orgasm difficulties is the condition called retarded ejaculation. Here, the male can attain high degrees of arousal, fully firm erections, and full participation in intercourse or other forms of sexual stimulation. His penis cooperates wonderfully up to this point in the response cycle. But men with retarded ejaculation have persistent difficulty reaching a climax. It is as though such men get stuck in the arousal phase of sexual response, unable to progress to orgasm. This condition may sound heavenly to a man who suffers from quick ejaculation, but such is not the case. Retarded ejaculation is typically quite frustrating, both to the men who suffer it and to their spouses.

Comparable to the male condition of retarded ejaculation is *female orgasmic dysfunction*. Here, a woman is able to become highly aroused and experience vaginal lubrication and swelling, but she is unable to experience orgasmic release with any form of sexual stimulation. Some women are able to achieve orgasm from self-stimulation but not from any form of stimulation by a partner.

Many women and their male partners mistakenly assume that the only healthy form of female sexual response is experiencing orgasm in response to penile-vaginal stimulation of the sort that typically occurs during intercourse. The truth is that most women do *not* experience orgasm from intercourse stimulation. For most women to achieve orgasm, they must receive sufficient stimulation of the clitoris, the tiny sexual organ located above the vaginal opening. Most of a woman's sexually pleasurable nerve endings are located in the clitoris, not in the vagina. A penis moving in and out of a vagina does not provide enough clitoral stimulation for most women to progress to orgasm. The majority of women who do report regularly experiencing orgasm during intercourse typically describe, if interviewed carefully, a pattern of lovemaking that involves receiving rather direct clitoral stimulation. It is this clitoral stimulation, not the stimulation from penile-vaginal contact, that usually triggers orgasm for most women.

With these sexual facts in mind, it is important for you and your partner to be realistic in your sexual expectations. A perfectly normal and healthy variation of female sexual response occurs when a woman enjoys lovemaking that involves intercourse but has orgasmic response only to oral or manual clitoral stimulation.

Vaginismus and Dyspareunia

Two specifically female sexual problems are *vaginismus* and *dyspareunia*. These problems do not involve direct physical shutdown of any single aspect of the sexual response cycle, but they are nonetheless quite painful and frustrating.

Vaginismus is a condition in which the muscles in the outer one-third of the vaginal canal automatically spasm in reaction to any attempted vaginal penetration. This condition can vary in severity. Some women experience vaginal tightening during attempted intercourse. This proves to be uncomfortable for both partners and makes intromission (insertion of the penis into the vagina) difficult to attain. Other women experience vaginal spasms so severe that no degree of intromission is possible. Such women even have difficulty undergoing a pelvic medical examination and often find it impossible because the vaginal muscles have developed a conditioned spasm reaction to any attempts at penetration.

Vaginal spasms can often be reconditioned so that pelvic exams and intercourse are possible. Treatment for this condition typically involves learning relaxation techniques, which are used in conjunction with gradually inserting one's own fingers, or vaginal dilators of progressively larger diameters. However, some women do not experience improvement from this technique because their vaginal spasm is rooted in discomfort that is caused by physical, not psychological, factors. These factors might involve infection, a vaginal lesion, uterine pain experienced during sexual arousal, or thinning of vaginal walls secondary to aging. For such women, relaxed vaginal musculature may be possible, but pain during intercourse, or dyspareunia, may be present. Dyspareunia can be caused by psychological factors, but this condition most often signals the existence of some physical problem. The specific nature and location of pain during intercourse can provide valuable information in diagnosing the cause of dyspareunia. Does the pain occur only during deep penile penetration, or immediately upon shallow penetration? Is pain limited only to certain intercourse positions? Once lubrication occurs, does the pain lessen? The answers to these questions help a physician to accurately diagnose the cause of dyspareunia and thus to treat the condition most effectively.

If you are experiencing either vaginismus or dyspareunia, it is especially important to have a thorough gynecological examination before attempting any behavioral or psychological forms of treatment. I recommend that you seek a thorough medical evaluation as a first step in dealing with *any* sexual performance difficulties, and this recommendation is strongest with reference to these two conditions.

Correcting Sexual Performance Problems

So now you understand the various things that can go wrong in your sex life. The question, of course, is, What can be done about this?

Treatment for any sexual performance problem can involve specific therapeutic interventions, but much of the treatment for each of these conditions is based on the foundation concepts explained in the following pages. Even if you are not regularly experiencing sexual performance problems, the following comments should prove quite helpful in improving your sexual relationship.

In discussing your sexual relationship with each other, I encourage you to remember that you are dealing with an important and complex topic, one that probably carries with it many feelings of vulnerability for each of you. Remember that sexual relating involves an intimate interplay of many aspects of your physical, emotional, and relationship patterns. When the specter of heart disease is added to this picture, things get even more complex. Improving your sex life therefore necessarily involves problem solving on multiple levels.

In organizing your efforts to enhance your sexual relating, it is helpful to understand and discuss your own and your partner's sexual responsivity from the following vantage points: biology, behavior, emotions, sexual beliefs, relationship styles, personality dynamics, and sensory experiences.

Biology

Contrary to popular beliefs, concerns about "safe sex" did not begin with the onset of the AIDS epidemic of the 1980s. Heart patients and their mates have long been plagued by the question of whether sexual activity and sexual response are physically safe.

Many cardiac couples stop having sex out of dread that the heart patient might die from the physical exertion involved in lovemaking. Other couples are so worried by this fear of death that they reduce their pattern of lovemaking to a brief and anxiety-laden form of biological release. In so doing, they deny themselves the intimacy and playfulness that sexual fulfillment should involve. For still other couples, sexual fulfillment and enjoyment diminish in the months and years following illness because of ignorance; they misunderstand the sexual consequences of medications and aging.

Let us look more closely at each of these issues—physical strain, aging, and medication—as they relate to sex and heart illness.

Sex and the Cardiovascular System

Pleasure during lovemaking will be ruined if you attend too much to distracting thoughts, worries, or noneroticbodily sensations. This fact applies to everyone, whether they have heart disease or not. Unfortunately, heart patients are especially likely to ruin their own sexual pleasure by overfocusing on their body symptoms. They notice their quickened heart rate, their shallow breathing, and the sound of their heartbeats as they are attempting to make love. They notice all this, but they forget to notice their feelings of sexual pleasure.

It is as though heart patients learn to fear that the physical signals of sexual arousal, such as increased heart rate and shallow breathing, are actually signs of an approaching heart attack. Further, they act as though they can ward off another heart attack if they closely monitor the inner workings of their cardiovascular system: "If I keep close enough watch on my heart's activities, it won't quit on me."

It is important to realize that sexual arousal does result in cardiovascular changes. As you become aroused, your heart pumps extra blood into your genitals, your heart rate speeds up a bit, and your blood pressure may rise somewhat. These cardiovascular events signal sexual arousal, not an upcoming heart attack. Even when you were seventeen years old and became sexually aroused, your heart rate sped up, your breathing got more shallow, and you could hear your heart pounding in your ears.

Now that you have become aware of heart illness, you have understandably become more sensitized to and bothered by the actions of your heart in many situations that require physical exertion—not just during sex. If you overfocus on your heart during sex, however, your worrying will interfere with your ability to respond sexually. Such monitoring of your heart will simply make you anxious; anxiety short-circuits sexual response and probably does nothing to improve anyone's heart condition, anyway.

As you gain confidence in your ability to tolerate physical exercise of various sorts, your worry about your cardiac response during sex should diminish. This worry is nicely soothed by educating yourself and your partner with the following facts about the relatively low amount of cardiac strain that is actually involved in sexual response.

The measure of the body's capacity for tolerating physical exertion that is typically used in cardiac rehabilitation settings is called the MET, which stands for metabolic energy testing. Through treadmill testing, the amount of oxygen your body uses during exertion can be expressed in the form of a MET level, a numerical rating of the heart's ability to manage comfortably the work involved in a given physical act. For example, 1 MET is equal to the amount of oxygen your body consumes while at rest. Cleaning windows requires 3–4 METs, digging a garden involves 5–6 METs, and digging ditches requires a 7–8 MET capacity.

Now here's the good news. Most middle-aged heart patients who have experienced uncomplicated heart attacks have an exercise capacity of 6–12 METs. Yet sexual response requires much less MET capacity than this. The energy expended during foreplay and afterplay requires approximately 3.5 METs, and orgasm requires a 4.7–5.5 METs capacity. In other words, for most people enjoyable lovemaking is no more dangerous than planting a garden!

Blood pressure and heart rate do increase during sexual response, but these increases are clearly within a safe range for most individuals. The average heart rate during lovemaking is 117 beats per minute, and a range of 90–144 beats is considered typical. Blood pressure increases to a maximum of 145/87 during a typical sexual encounter. These increases in heart rate and blood pressure last only briefly, and the body returns to a normal baseline level of cardiac exertion rather quickly after orgasm.

All these measures of cardiac response tend to improve (that is, to lessen) as general physical conditioning improves. So if you are having trouble motivating yourself to exercise regularly to rehabilitate your heart, exercise so that you can begin making love better and with less strain and stress.

A small percentage of heart patients do experience irregular heartbeats during sexual arousal, more likely because sexual response involves a unique emotional aspect than because of any direct cardiac problem. The emotional intensity of arousal triggers certain sympathetic nervous system actions, which, in part, also trigger heart arrhythmias. For other people, sexual interaction, like many other forms of exercise, triggers angina.

If you are having cardiac symptoms during sex, discuss them with your doctor. If the doctor assures you that you are not experiencing any particular cardiac complications from sexual response, try making the following behavioral changes:

- Learn to relax and focus on sexual arousal, not on your heart.
- Be sure that you are physically comfortable while having sex. Use sexual positions that allow you to relax your arm and chest muscles.
- Try having sex during times when you are generally fresh and relaxed, like in the mornings.
- With your doctor's permission, you might try taking nitro-glycerin before lovemaking, to alleviate distracting cardiac symptoms.

Now your fears about whether sex is safe should be allayed. However, two other factors—medication and age—must also be understood so that you can continue to manage this very important aspect of your marriage and of the cardiac rehabilitation process.

Sex and Medication

There is no doubt that many medications have negative effects on sexual response. Some medicines affect sex drive, some inhibit arousal, and some impair orgasm or ejaculation.

The difficulty is that it is impossible to predict which medication will affect a given individual in which sexual ways. For example, if ten men are given the same blood pressure medication at the same dosage level, some may experience impaired erection while others may notice no sexual side effects whatsoever. The probable reason why reactions to medication differ is that everyone's body interacts somewhat uniquely with any chemical that is ingested. This is obvious from the different ways we all react to such drugs as caffeine, nicotine, and alcohol.

Psychological expectation—what you think will happen—can also have much to do with the sexual side effects of medication. It has been said that the chief sexual organ in the body is the brain. Various research studies have documented that expecting a given medication or drug to have a given sexual effect, either positive or negative, can sometimes produce the effect, even when the "drug" is a placebo (for example, a sugar pill, or a drink that smells like alcohol but actually contains none).

For these reasons, making absolute statements about the sexual effects of various medicines is difficult. However, it is possible to offer some general guidelines about the sexual changes that may occur with various heart medicines.

Of most concern are the blood pressure medications. Many high blood pressure medicines negatively affect sexual response. Heart patients are often confused about why this happens. It seems logical to assume that because these medicines lower blood pressure, they must also lessen the heart's ability to pump blood into the body's sexual areas. One patient complained, "This medicine has slowed my heart down so much that it just can't pump fast enough to keep up with my sexual thoughts and feelings." This is not really accurate. The interference of these medicines on sexual response is due to a neurological effect, not to a blood flow effect. These drugs block the neurological reflex arc that is part of the body's sexual response cycle. They do not weaken your heart or its ability to pump blood.

As Saul Rosenthal explains in his excellent book, *Sex over Forty*,[4] there are five main classes of high blood pressure medicines, each of which carries certain risks of potential sexual side effects. The research on the sexual risks associated with each of the five major classes of antihypertensive medications is summarized in table 8.1.

1. The diuretics work by increasing the excretion of salt and water through urine. These are probably the most widely used antihypertensive medicines, and they are generally found to have minimal or no negative sexual side effects. The one diuretic that has been found to have predictable negative sexual side effects is Aldactone, which decreases the level of testosterone in men if administered at high doses. This lowering of testosterone can cause impotence, breast enlargement, and loss of sex drive. Fortunately, this particular diuretic is used only rarely these days in the treatment of high blood pressure.

[4]S. Rosenthal, *Sex over Forty* (Los Angeles: Jeremy P. Tarcher, 1987).

Table 8.1 Sexual Side Effects of Antihypertensive Medications

Medication Type	Brand Names	Possible Sexual Side Effects
Diuretics	Aldactone Dyazide Enduron Esidrex Hydro-Diuril Hygroton Lasix Maxzide Naqua Oretic	Minimal or none, except Aldactone, which may cause impotence and loss of sex drive.
Sympathetic blockers	Aldomet Blocadren Catapres Corgard Inderal Ismelin Lopressor Reserpine Serpasil Tenormin Trandate	At high dosages problems include lessened sex drive, erection and ejaculation problems (for men), and impaired orgasm (for women). Fewest sexual side effects are from Corgard, Tenormin, and Trandate.
Vasodilators	Apresoline Minipress	None.
Calcium channel blockers	Calan Cardizem Isoptin Procardia	None.
ACE inhibitors	Capoten Vasotec	None.

Source: Adapted from Saul H. Rosenthal, M.D., *Sex over Forty* (Los Angeles: Jeremy P. Tarcher, 1987), pp. 164–68.

2. The sympathetic blockers work by blocking certain types of nerve cell receptors. These medicines include the beta blockers, the alpha and beta blockers, and others. In general, these widely used antihypertensives do tend to interfere with full sexual responsivity. Fairly recent advances in these medicines have diminished this trait, but high doses of the sympathetic blockers usually lead to negative sexual side effects.

Lower doses are less likely to interfere with sexual response. (This fact should further motivate you to control your blood pressure by attending to diet, weight, and exercise aspects of your life-style.)

Again, there are no absolute predictions regarding the effects of these medicines. Inderol, Lopressor, and Reserpine tend to cause depression and corresponding lessening of sexual drive. Aldomet is probably the most documented culprit of this group with regard to negative sexual side effects. Up to 40 percent of patients report loss of sexual desire, inability to ejaculate (for men), and impaired orgasm (for women) when taking high doses of Aldomet. Ismelin, too, has been found to inhibit ejaculation in a high percentage of men. Catapres has been found to inhibit erection and ejaculation in 10 to 20 percent of men taking it, to impair orgasm in women, and to lower sex drive in both sexes. Tenormin, Corgard, and Trandate appear to be the best choices among the sympathetic blockers with regard to lessened risk of sexual side effects. However, it is important to emphasize the great degree of individual difference in response to all these medications. The important point is to discover *your* reaction to a given medication.

3. The third group of antihypertensives, the *vasodilators,* are rarely used alone in controlling high blood pressure because advances have been made in effectiveness of other classes of drugs, such as the calcium channel blockers and the ACE inhibitors. The two brands of vasodilators most frequently prescribed are Apresoline and Minipress. Neither has been found to have many negative effects on sexual functioning.

4. The *calcium channel blockers* are a new group of medicines that are used in treating both arrhythmia and high blood pressure. The calcium channel blockers rarely cause any sexual side effects. Unfortunately, these medicines are helpful to only about one person in three in controlling blood pressure.

5. The newest group of antihypertensives, the *angiotensin-converting enzyme inhibitors* (or *ACE inhibitors),* have virtually

no negative side effects, including effect on sexual activity.
This is rapidly becoming the most frequently prescribed
group of blood pressure medicines.

In general, it is clear that most people experience no negative sexual side effects from most antihypertensive medications. Even medicines that have been documented as having negative effects on sexual functioning affected a minority, not a majority, of the patients sampled.

It is also clear that there are many different types of blood pressure medicines. If you are having negative side effects from any medication, you should consult your physician about the possibility of trying another medicine or a different dosage level of the same one.

Some physicians are not responsive to patients' concerns about sexual side effects of medication. They convey the impression that the sexual impairment is minor or that sexual impairment is of less concern than the need to control blood pressure. It might be helpful to remind such a doctor that the only minor sexual problem is one that is happening to someone else; in your own sex life, impairment is a major concern! No one would disagree that controlling blood pressure is more crucial to overall health than having full sexual response. But it is also important to remember that there are many antihypertensive medications from which to choose. A different medication might very well control your blood pressure and have no negative effect on your sex life.

It is important to be realistic and honest with yourself about this issue. I frequently treat heart patients who have so many factors operating in their lives that could diminish sexual response that specifying the particular effects of antihypertensive medication is impossible. These factors might include excessive weight, blockage of blood flow to the pelvic area because of hardening of arteries, nicotine or alcohol abuse, excessive stress, marital tensions, the effects of other medications (such as antidepressants, antihistamines, or ulcer medications), and the normal effects of the aging process. As a first step in deciding whether to try a new medication, most physicians wisely recommend that you change any of these factors that are changeable. Only then will you be able to make a reasonable judgment as to whether your sexual problems are being caused by your medication.

Sex and Aging

We generally make one of two possible mistakes in our assumptions about the sexual changes of growing older: we either underestimate or overestimate the effect that the normal aging process has on sexual response. The fact is that clear and predictable changes in sexual responsivity begin as early as the mid-thirties. This certainly does not mean that you are over the sexual hill by your fortieth birthday; enjoyable and effective sexual response can be maintained throughout your life. However, it is essential that you and your mate be realistic and sensible about the facts of sex and aging.

The physical changes that come with age do not necessarily cause sexual performance problems. However, as can be seen in the example of Glenn and Lois, sexual problems do often result from anxiety caused by uneducated reactions to the sexual aging process.

Glenn was fifty-two years old and his wife, Lois, was fifty-seven. Glenn had undergone coronary bypass surgery at age forty-eight and had recuperated with no physical complications. Glenn's contact with me came after Lois was referred for help with depression. Her referring physician assumed that Lois's sad mood, withdrawn behavior, and general lack of zest were related to the empty nest syndrome created by the relatively recent marriage of her only child.

As I got to know this couple, several things quickly became clear. The marriage of their daughter certainly did begin a new phase of life for Glenn and Lois; they loved being parents, and they missed their former close contact with their only child. However, the empty nest had little to do with Lois's depression. More bothersome to her, marital intimacy had steadily dwindled in the preceding three years. She and Glenn had once been openly affectionate and spontaneously loving in their relationship. Now their marriage had turned into a relationship of tense distancing and avoidance of physical touch.

The difficulties began when they noticed that Glenn, who had typically been the sexual pursuer in the relationship, began having less firm and less spontaneous erections. In the past, Glenn could become aroused and erect merely in reaction to the sight of his wife dressing or undressing. Beginning around age fifty, however, both partners noticed that Glenn required rather prolonged manual or oral stimulation of his penis by Lois before he could get fully erect.

This absolutely normal change in sexual responsivity frightened and confused this couple. Lois quietly wondered if her long-standing fear of losing her attractiveness to her younger husband was finally justified now. Glenn began to obsess about his fear that the athero-sclerosis that had resulted in his need for coronary bypass surgery might now be blocking blood flow to his penis.

All this quiet worry and fear led to mutual tension about sex. This loving and open couple became progressively more withdrawn from each other and began avoiding the topic of sex. They soon became caught in a vicious cycle: the more they quietly worried, the more they avoided sex and physical affection. The more they avoided, the more anxious and worried they became. As they both became more anx-ious, sex drive and sexual response were further squelched for both of them. In addition to distancing physically, each began to assume that the other was being quietly critical. Tension and irritability replaced their typical comfort when they attempted to communicate.

Subtly and progressively, what had been a healthy, intimate mar-riage deteriorated into a relationship between two lonely and anxious people. Like many couples, Lois and Glenn were caught in the unfor-tunate trap of discomfort that results from misunderstanding the natu-ral changes in sexual response that occur as the body ages.

The tragedy of the story of Glenn and Lois is that their difficulties would never have occurred if they had had a clear and realistic under-standing of the basic facts about sex and the aging process. Knowing what to expect as the natural result of aging would have prevented the problems that were now threatening their happiness.

The main fact to remember about sex and aging is that, *as we age, we need more direct and more prolonged stimulation of our sexual body areas in order to progress through the sexual response cycle.* It is as though the hormonal changes that happen for both men and women beginning around age thirty-five result in a prolongation of the sexual response cycle. Whereas you used to be able to progress rapidly from non-arousal to arousal to orgasm, it is likely that you will need to be more patient, attentive, and physically loving of each other as age diminishes sexual hormones and slows your sexual responsivity.

As they age, men require more direct and more lengthy stimulation of the penis to get erect. Furthermore, the erection may not be quite as full or as hard as in prior years. Correspondingly, aging women may require more direct and more lengthy stimulation of the breasts and clitoral area to become aroused. There may also be less vaginal lubrication during arousal than in prior years. Once aroused, both men and women require increased direct stimulation of the sexual areas to trigger orgasm as age advances. The orgasm response may be somewhat less intense than in younger years—very relaxing and satisfying, but less explosive.

To understand sex and aging, it is helpful to understand the effects that hormones have on both male and female sexual response. The effects of the male hormone testosterone were discussed in the Sex Drive section. As the testosterone level drops with each advancing decade past age thirty-five, sexual responsivity slows down in the ways just described. But even though the level of this hormone diminishes as we age, our sexual hormones do not disappear. Most men and women continue to have ample testosterone to fuel sexual response throughout life.

The sexual consequences of aging are somewhat more complicated for women because of the abrupt hormonal changes that occur during menopause. During menopause (which typically occurs sometime around age fifty), there is a sudden decrease in the primary female sex hormone, estrogen. Decreased estrogen does not directly lessen sex drive, arousal, or orgasm response in women. It is therefore often said that there is no physical reason for a woman's sex life to be negatively affected by menopause.

The hormonal changes that occur in menopause do create various physical side effects, however, which may affect female sexual response. Because estrogen is the hormone that fuels the development of female sexual organs, the long-term effects of lowered levels of this hormone include physical changes in the vagina. These changes include a gradual thinning of the vaginal walls and a subsequent loss of vaginal elasticity and cushioning. The result is a narrowing of the vaginal opening. Losing estrogen also results in a lessening of vaginal lubrication during sexual arousal. This combination of lessened va-

ginal lubrication and elasticity can result in discomfort during intercourse unless additional lubrication is used. Such lubricants include
surgical jellies (like K-Y Jelly), Albolene Cream, and Lubrin.

Many women going through menopause are treated with estrogen replacement therapy to lessen the uncomfortable symptoms of
this period of hormonal changing. A combination of estrogen and progestin is prescribed in order to mimic the body's former cycle of hormonal secretion, and symptoms such as hot flashes, irritability, and
vaginal changes are thus diminished.

Estrogen replacement therapy was originally thought to increase
the risks of breast and uterine cancer and to pose particular risks for
women suffering from hypertension or heart illness. However, current
medical thought seems to be that, when properly prescribed and
taken, this is a relatively safe and effective therapy for virtually all
menopausal women, including those suffering from heart illness. I
strongly recommend that you consult your gynecologist about this option. Most menopausal women report significant improvements in
overall quality of life and enhanced sexual enjoyment as a result of
estrogen replacement therapy.

It is obviously true that aging does, indeed, affect sexual responsiveness. However, the good news is that we maintain our ability to
respond sexually throughout our lives, particularly if we continue
to exercise our sexual organs. Men and women in their sixties and sev-
enties respond more fully to sexual stimulation if they maintain patterns of regular sexual response, either through lovemaking or through
masturbation. In other words, the best way to keep from losing it is to
keep using it.

Advancing age also typically brings increased maturity, wisdom,
and relationship security. These factors should lead to increased flexibility in your attitudes toward sex. Expand your perspective from the
narrow notion that sex has to do only with an erect penis inside a lubricated vagina. Think of your sexual relationship with the freeing notion that lovemaking has to do with orchestrating a whole symphony
of intimacy containing many movements, variations on the themes of
affection and communication, and intimate behaviors. With this ex-
pansion of attitude comes the stuff that makes a better sex life.

Even though your body changes in the direction of some slowing of the sexual response as you age, remember my prior comment: The body's largest sexual organ is the brain. Understanding the facts about sex and aging should help you develop and maintain a soothing attitude about this aspect of life.

So how is your sex life, from a biological perspective? If you suspect or know that some physical or chemical factor is negatively affecting your sexual response, don't give up; get more information about your condition and the possible medical treatments available to you. Recent medical advances have made possible the accurate evaluation and successful treatment of many organically caused sexual problems. Pelvic angiography can assess the degree of circulation to the pelvic area. It is also possible to determine penile blood pressure as a means of evaluating whether a biological problem underlies erection difficulties.

Medical aids can enhance blood flow to the penis, and surgical procedures can often restore or aid sexual response. One such procedure involves grafting new blood flow pathways to the penis to aid erection. Another surgery involves the insertion of a penile prosthesis into the penile cavities to allow for the simulation of a natural erection. These surgeries are safe, medically sound, and most often effective in enhancing the sex life of any partners who are otherwise open and loving in their efforts to maintain intimate connections through all the years of their life together.

Behavior

The second major factor to consider in evaluating and communicating about your sex life is behavior. Two questions apply here: (1) Are you orchestrating your sexual interactions in a way that is cardiovascularly sensible? (2) Are you being sexually sensible in your lovemaking encounters?

Most heart patients experience some form of cardiac symptomatology at some points during lovemaking. It is also true that most people who suffer from arthritis experience arthritic pain sometimes during lovemaking, that many people who have ulcers sometimes notice a stomachache during sex, and so on. The big difference here is that heart patients and their spouses *fear* these occasional flare-ups of their health problems. The big fear lurking in the bedrooms of many cardiac couples is that someone might die during sex. Both the heart patient and the spouse typically harbor at least fleeting thoughts of this sort.

Just in case you were not adequately soothed by the facts I reported about the physical safety of sexual exertion, I will now add another fact to your arsenal of coping tools: Death during intercourse from a coital coronary is an extremely rare phenomenon.

An often-cited research study in the cardiac literature found that of the sudden deaths that were recorded in the year of investigation, less than one-tenth of 1 percent involved a heart patient dying from a heart attack experienced during lovemaking.[5] Furthermore—and most important—similar studies have found that approximately 80 percent of the individuals who suffer coital coronaries do so while having sex late in the evening after hours of heavy eating and heavy alcohol consumption, and while having sex with someone other than their spouses. The moral of this research is obvious: Behave yourself! Messing around can kill you.

It should now be obvious that, from a cardiac standpoint, sex is safe. Using common sense is all that is required to behaviorally manage any cardiac concerns about sex. Just treat sex like a very special and enjoyable form of exercise. Make choices about when and how to engage in this form of exercise just as you do with other forms of physical exertion.

After all, you know better than to exercise in excessive heat or cold, or when you are fatigued or bogged down from a recent meal. You probably find exercising easier in the morning after a restful night's sleep than in the late evening after a long and tiring day. When choosing your type of exercise, you probably choose something that suits both your tastes and your physical capabilities. You probably avoid forms of exercise that require you to put your body in painful or excessively stressful positions.

On your doctor's recommendation, you might even take nitroglycerin before exercising, to ward off exertional angina. If you do ex-

[5]M. Ueno, The so-called coition death, *Japanese Journal of Legal Medicine* 17 (1963): 333–40.

perience chest pains or atypical shortness of breath during exercising, you probably slow your pace, change activities, or simply stop and rest awhile. After exercising, you probably allow yourself a recovery and resting period. This allows you both to recuperate physically and to enjoy for a moment the good feelings that have come from your body's release of energy.

Are these descriptions of sensible rules for exercising referring to walking, swimming, jogging, or sexual intercourse? The answer, of course, is yes.

It is important to discover, by experimenting with time and place and by talking openly with each other, what forms of sexual relating in which situations are most comfortable for each of you. By so clarifying, you will be able to relax and enjoy the pleasuring at hand and put out of your bedroom (or whichever room you like) any distracting anxieties about cardiac complications from sexual exertion.

Once your concerns about heart symptoms are put aside, you can then concentrate your efforts on being good lovers for each other. To do so, you must take responsibility for learning and teaching each other about effective lovemaking. You must discover your partner's sexual likes and dislikes and learn to provide the forms of loving stimulation that are especially pleasurable for your partner and acceptable to you. And you must learn what your own sexual pleasures are and take responsibility for teaching your partner to be a good lover for you.

Remember, you greatly increase the odds that your sexual needs will be met if you accurately identify and clearly express these needs in a loving and appropriate manner. Being a good lover does not mean knowing what your partner wants; it means knowing how to find out what your partner wants, and being willing to give generously in this very special way. Let each other know what these special sexual gifts might be.

Emotions

Now that you are unafraid of sex, understand your own biology, and are getting the right amounts of the right kinds of sexual stimulation, you are ready for the fun to begin! All you need to respond sexually is to remain relaxed.

Relaxation is one of the most crucial ingredients in the formula for effective sexual response. If you are experiencing anything other than comfortable relaxation while having sex, the odds increase that your body will turn off the sexual response cycle and turn on some other emotional or physical set of responses. This is particularly true if you are experiencing any antierotic emotions such as fear, anger, apprehension, anxiety, or frustration. When you experience such feelings, your body sends blood to places other than your sexual organs.

A complicating factor in the sex life of any cardiac couple is that painful emotions do occur as part of coping with heart illness. It is perfectly normal to feel anxious, afraid, depressed, and angry occasionally during cardiac rehabilitation. It is to be hoped, though, that you will not become stuck in any such negative emotion. If you do, more than your sex life will suffer, and you should get professional help in learning to understand and cope better with the worries that face you.

You must accept that attempting to perform sexually while feeling negative emotions is not likely to prove very pleasurable or successful, particularly after age thirty-five. In earlier years you were so filled with hormones (relatively speaking) that your biology could perhaps override your emotions, and full sexual response could occur no matter how you felt emotionally. This does not remain the case as we mature. Attempting to soothe jangled nerves by having sex is not a good idea. It simply increases the odds that you will soon have something new to worry about: difficulty becoming aroused or experiencing orgasm.

It takes only a few such episodes of failed sexual performance before the very thought of making love begins to stir feelings of discomfort. Then the self-defeating, vicious circle of sexual "spectatoring" begins. Soon it seems as if four people are attempting to make love whenever you and your partner are in bed: you, your mate, a part of you standing at bedside evaluating how you are doing, and a part of your mate standing at bedside worrying that you might get upset if you do not respond perfectly.

What a lot of pressure! This process of spectatoring is a major culprit in perpetuating sexual performance problems. It is important to learn to relax and get out of your head and into your senses so that you can begin enjoying your natural sexual responsiveness again. To do so, it is helpful, first, to examine whether you are talking yourself into dysfunction-producing sexual anxiety and, second, to learn to focus on sensory sensations and imagery to combat that anxiety.

Sexual Beliefs

In chapter 14, I discuss extensively the interplay between thoughts and emotions, emphasizing how what you think affects the way you feel. Here, I want to underscore the importance of this notion in managing your sexual response. It is important to learn consciously to control your thinking habits (your "self talk") in evaluating your sexual abilities. Heart patients are especially prone to make three anxiety-producing thinking errors in evaluating and anticipating their sexual responsiveness:

1. *Overgeneralizing.* Some create performance anxiety and despair by overreacting to any fluctuations in sexual response. Example: "I couldn't get an erection last night, so I guess this heart attack has left me impotent forever."

2. *Personalizing blame.* Others demoralize themselves and perpetuate further fear of failure by fueling guilt with self-blame. Example: "First I turn this family upside down with this heart attack, and now I don't even have any sex drive. I know my husband can't take much more of my problems. He looks sad and mad half the time and I know it's my fault."

3. *All-or-nothing evaluations.* Still others perpetuate self-defeating sexual pressures by convincing themselves that if things are not going perfectly, then a catastrophe is at hand. Example: "Oh no! Here we are naked, she's all turned on and romantic, and I'm not as hard as I usually get. This is never going to work! If I can't get it all the way up, I know she'll notice and be upset. Why even try if this is all I can do?"

Of course, there is no limit to the various ways you can fuss and shame yourself when sexual faltering occurs. Being judgmental and feeling insecure in evaluating your sexual performance seems inevitable, in view of the unrealistic standards that we are taught to use as yardsticks for measuring our own sexual styles and capabilities.

In his book, *Male Sexuality,*[6] Bernie Zilbergeld makes the point that movies and pornographic and romantic literature would have us believe some rather interesting stuff about what is sexually normal. Those images might make us feel inadequate if we differ from them in any way. For example, men might believe that only a very large penis can satisfy a woman, and women might believe that men find only large breasts exciting. These media-contrived images are false. Sexual tastes vary, which means there is no one ideal. We can watch pornographic movies and read pornographic literature, but we should never measure ourselves—our appearance or our performance—by the actors and characters who appear there.

We all compare ourselves with these ridiculous standards of sexual performance to some degree, and the comparisons inevitably make us feel inadequate and self-conscious. With this backdrop, we are clearly set up to overreact if the consequences of aging and heart disease result in real sexual performance difficulties.

One of the many ways we torture ourselves sexually is by assuming that our partner really wants and expects the movie version of sexual interaction that we know we cannot provide. Worry and apprehension result, at least, and perhaps resentment too, all because of what may be an unfounded assumption about what your partner really wants. Rather than assume, try asking. It is far wiser and infinitely more healing to speak openly and honestly with each other about your sexual expectations, hopes, dreams, fears, and impressions of each other. To do so will normally soothe any fear-generating assumptions about what your partner wants sexually.

One delightful patient of mine once said to her worried heart patient husband: "If you came home one day preceded by a 'throbbing organ' that was leaping out at me and all over the room, I would jump out the window. Sexual athletes are okay to watch in the movies, but when it comes time for *me* to get naked, I want to do it with someone who isn't going to scare me to death and make me feel inadequate with his sexual acrobatics."

[6]B. Zilbergeld, *Male Sexuality* (New York: Bantam Books, 1978).

Realistic and honest sharing helps to quiet unrealistc, anxiety-generating thinking. Picture yourself in your mind's eye and describe yourself in your inner voice as being someone who comfortably and effectively engages in lovemaking with your partner. Your body will cooperate with the images and dialogue that guide it.

Relationship Styles

The creation of sexual intimacy depends ultimately on the most basic of relationship factors—cooperation. A solo attempt to create sexual intimacy is like trying to clap with only one hand; the essential other ingredient in the formula is missing. The best way to soothe sexual performance concerns is to cooperate in creating and maintaining a loving and communicative relationship. Nothing squelches sexual response quicker than relationship tension.

In examining your sexual relationship, remember my prior comments about marriage partners working as teams that organize around and are affected by the emotional themes that predominate in the relationship. Changes in sexual response can signal unresolved relationship problems. And if your changes in sexual response are caused by factors other than the relationship itself, unresolved relationship problems will interfere with your making a positive adjustment to those sexual changes.

As I have repeatedly stated, your sexual response changes as you age and in reaction to momentary states such as stress, fatigue, anxiety, or any of the many factors mentioned in this chapter. What happens *next* in your relationship determines your ultimate sexual adjustment.

If you and your partner are locked into uncomfortable patterns of reacting to your sexual changes, you must lovingly cooperate in order to change. Try reading together the preceding sections in this book on healthy marriages (chapter 4), intimacy building (chapter 7), and sexuality. Open and expand your styles of communicating with each other, both verbally and physically. Experiment by changing your overall relationship patterns, not just in the bedroom, but in your general style of relating to each other:

If you are typically quiet, start talking.

If you typically hold back when hugged, start hugging back.

If you usually criticize, find something to compliment.

If you usually wait for your partner to initiate physical affection, switch roles.

If you are in the boring habit of silently watching television after dinner, take a walk and hold hands as you talk.

Behaving differently often leads to feeling different in a relationship. Try it; you have nothing to lose and much pleasure to gain.

If you repeatedly find that some negative emotional reaction to each other interferes with your attempts to build intimacy, perhaps you would be helped by a brief course of professional marital counseling. Put aside any outdated stigma that you may associate with counseling. Seeking professional guidance in dealing with a complicated issue is an intelligent, healthy, and loving choice to make. You deserve this much.

Personality Dynamics

Sex means different things to different people, depending on their personality makeup. For some, sexual relating is a duty to perform as part of a relationship contract. For others, sexual release is a primary form of relaxation to counter accumulated life pressures. Still others cling desperately to sexual interaction as a source of validation of personal worth and attractiveness. Sex is a brief and goal-directed performance for some and a meandering, playful give-and-take for others.

The way we react sexually is often an indicator of our gut-level psychological action. Pay attention to each other and to yourself in this regard. If your sexual pattern of interaction has changed or if your inner feeling about sex is one of discomfort, perhaps you are being affected by some unresolved aspect of your personality-based reactions to sexual intimacy or to the overall stresses of the rehabilitation process.

For example, some people are programmed to feel discomfort with intimacy in general. They feel most comfortable staying at a physical and emotional arm's length from other people. Others are programmed to feel comfortable with intimacy as long as interactions remain nonsexual. Such people typically associate some antierotic emotion such as guilt, fear, shame, or anxiety with open sexual expression.

Both personality-based reactions and stresses of rehabilitation were probably affecting one of my extremely time-urgent, anxious, Type A heart patients, who once bragged to me, "I haven't slowed down a bit since my heart attack. My wife and I have sex at least three times a week."

His wife replied, "Since his heart attack, everything about him has speeded up, including his sex life. We do have sex three times a week—for a total of about six minutes. He gets on me, then gets off me. It's as though he's running from something and is afraid to slow down. He's always been hard driving, but he's never been as unaware as he is now."

Still other personalities have no particular difficulty feeling permission to enjoy sexual intimacy; they have an accurate and educated understanding of what it takes to have a good sex life. Their problem is that they are exhausted by the stresses that are being fueled by their personality-based coping patterns. Being burned out with worry, fatigue, stress, or frustration is hardly any way to begin feeling sexy.

Exploring the many possible causes of and solutions to personality-based roots of sexual dysfunction is beyond the scope of this book. However, developing a basic understanding of each other's personality makeup can greatly help you control your reactions, both in responding sexually and in responding to illness. These topics are discussed in the following three chapters.

Let it suffice to say that if you and your partner are experiencing sexual struggle that does not improve when you try the various cognitive, behavioral, and relationship strategies outlined in this chapter, then perhaps basic differences in personality are at the root of your problems. This does not mean that you cannot change.

Openly communicating about these differences may help lessen your discomfort in this area. Or it may be necessary to receive professional psychological counseling to learn to overcome old anxieties that are interfering with your intimacy. In either case, it pays to believe in your own and your partner's ability to learn to relax and enjoy safe and comfortable sexual intimacy. Loving, patient support from each other is of great help in making such changes.

Sensory Experiences

The most effective way to enhance sexual pleasure is to enjoy your sexual response using all five of your senses: sight, smell, taste, hearing, and touch.

The most effective way to ruin your sexual fun is to fill your head with distracting and bothersome thoughts instead of sexual sensations. The classic way to defeat sexual pleasure is to repeatedly command yourself to stop worrying about your sexual response. This never works, because we are cognitively unable to process negative commands. Try this: *Do not* think about a white elephant. Now *do not* picture that white elephant's long, white trunk and floppy, white ears. *Do not* think about that white elephant's round, stumpy legs and enormous white elephant head. In order not to think about this image, you first have to picture it and then cognitively cross out awareness of the picture. In the process, guess what happened: you thought about the very thing you were trying to block out.

This is exactly what we do when we try to soothe ourselves about sexual anxieties by repeatedly reminding ourselves not to worry about performing during lovemaking. If we could hear and see a tape of what we run through our minds during lovemaking once we become anxious about our performance, it would probably go something like this:

"Okay, here we are, doing all right so far. Both half-naked, the lights are low, we're in the mood, all the right stuff is happening. I'm just *not* going to worry about whether my penis will show up for this performance—even though he sure has been on vacation a lot since my heart attack. I'm *not* going to worry about failing and disappointing my wife. I think I'll give her a little kiss. . . .

"Now, where was I? Oh yes, Old Faithful—he's not what he used to be, but I'm just *not* going to worry about the fact that he's only halfway hard tonight. Oh-oh! She's touching me down there. . . . Maybe she won't notice. I'd better keep still; if I move my hips, Old But Not So Faithful Anymore Since My Heart Attack might bend in her hand, and then she'll know. But I'm just not going to worry about what she's thinking about my half-hard penis. That's it. I'm just going to lie here and not worry about any of this stuff. . . . Oh, Lord, help me not worry about any of this. . . . "

Now, really. How many penises could stand up under that kind of pressure?

More effective and enjoyable than such torturous and misguided attempts *not* to worry is the strategy of filling your mind with so much pleasurable sexual sensory awareness that there is no room for worrying or not worrying.

Fortunately, most of us cannot consciously process more than seven pieces of information at once. You can use this fact to your sexual advantage by filling your mind with five chunks of sexual sensory information. Use each of the sensory channels to tune in to the sexual experience at hand, and you will greatly increase the odds that your body will respond with sexual pleasure. *Look* at your bodies as you are touching each other and making love to each other, or close your eyes and picture yourselves in your mind's eye. Notice the *smell* of your partner's skin or hair. *Feel* the warmth of your bodies coming together and the soothing and the unique combination of relaxation and excitement that happens during sexual arousal. *Listen* to the sexual sounds that you make together and exchange sexy and loving comments as you romance each other. Relish that familiar *taste* of your partner's mouth or shoulder as you caress. Fill your head with all this, and there will be no room for worrying.

Feeling somewhat anxious about making love is understandable following heart illness or following any prolonged period during which you have avoided sex. A loving and sensible way to bolster your ability to learn to relax and enjoy your sexual responses is to start from scratch and only gradually build up to full sexual involvement.

First, take time to practice tuning into your own bodily reactions to soothing touch, sexy thoughts, or sexy pictures. If you can, put aside any religious, moral, or emotional prohibitions that you may have against sexual self-stimulation. View this as a medical recommendation geared toward helping you regain confidence so that both your medical and relationship rehabilitation tasks can be addressed more successfully. Learn to become aroused, to lessen arousal by simply relaxing, and then to restimulate arousal.

Next, invite your partner to join you in relaxing sessions of sexual pleasuring. Free each other from any demands or expectations to "perform" during these pleasuring sessions. Agree not to have sexual intercourse for a while; these sessions are intended simply to be relaxing and soothing. Take turns massaging and caressing each other. Using warmed oils or lotions, give each other lengthy, loving, full-body massages, skipping your sexual body areas for now. While receiving this special attention, simply relax and tune in with all your senses. Then, with the same multisensory focus, lovingly massage your partner.

Once you have learned to remain reasonably relaxed during this form of loving interaction, you can begin to make your times together a little more erotic by incorporating manual or oral stimulation of each other's sexual areas. But *do not* turn this into pressure to perform sexually, either for yourself or for your partner. If you begin to feel distracted or tense, drop back a step and find the mode of interacting that is comfortable for you.

Gradually incorporate more specific erotic stimulation into these times of pleasuring each other. Use these massages as opportunities to expand your sexual comfort zones, both as individuals and as a couple. For example, it is very healthy and helpful to learn to feel comfortable making love to each other even if an erect penis and a lubricated vagina are not available during a particular lovemaking session. Remember, this is not a performance. Be loving, communicative, nurturing, and playful, and fill your mind with awareness of the sensations at hand.

Eventually, if you so desire, you might begin to incorporate controlled intercourse into these loving encounters. Take your time, notice yourselves as you make love. Avoid switching into any old anxiety-producing and intimacy-squelching ways of rushing or of demanding performance from self or other. Notice and appreciate your own and your partner's ability to create the experience of being on an island of refuge amid your overall life stresses. Get out of your minds and into your senses. By doing this together, you can enjoy your sexual relationship through all the days of your marriage.

Summary

To manage your sex life healthfully, remember these points:

In every couple, differences exist in sexual drive, sexual response patterns, and sexual preferences. These differences may become exaggerated by the stress of adjusting to illness.

It is normal to experience periodic difficulties in progressing through any of the phases of sexual response—arousal, plateau, and orgasm. Learn to relax and continue your loving involvement without obsessing about past "failures."

Responding sexually is certainly safe from a cardiovascular standpoint. But your sexual response may be altered by the effects of aging, of medication, or of your overall physical condition.

Regardless of your particular physical condition, you can enjoy the sexual aspect of your relationship more if you use common sense in controlling your behavioral, emotional, and thought patterns as you orchestrate your sex life.

Remember that sexual feelings are a by-product of personality-based modes of relating to others and of the relationship patterns that you create in your marriage.

By lovingly attending to this important aspect of life and marriage, you add a comforting and important factor to your overall cardiac rehabilitation process.

Your sex life has to do with more than just penis and vagina. It has to do with the interplay between your own and your partner's most intimate, most vulnerable, and most wonderful layers of that inner sense of self that houses your unique and special gifts.

By being open, caring, honest, playful, and sensible with each other, you can continue to improve the quality of your sexual relationship throughout your life together.

Part III

. . . . . .

The Personality Factor: Can We Change?

Nine

Personality

■ ■ ■ ■ ■ ■

*B*y this point, you may be saying, justifiably, "That's all fine and good, and it makes sense. Now we understand in more elaborate detail how we are as a couple—the good, the bad, and the ugly of it all. But so what? Being like this just comes naturally; it's just the way we are and always have been. Our personalities make us react in these ways, and our personalities aren't going to change just because we're now coping with illness."

Without doubt, there is a definite limit to how much we can change our personality-based coping patterns. We do seem to battle the same old feelings of low self-esteem and struggle with variations of the same old anxieties and fears from the time of grade school throughout adulthood. It is almost as though there is a part of us that simply will not be soothed by new information—a negative "inner sense of self" that is a constant source of painful and anxiety-generating reactions that continue to haunt us. Consider only a few examples of how some people continue to be plagued by earlier life experiences: Slender adults who were overweight as children still feel like fat people in disguise. Successful and powerful adults sometimes still feel driven by the quest to overcome the powerlessness they remember from the pain of always being chosen last when teams were picked on the playground. Hard-driving, competitive individuals who intimidate others often still feel the painful shyness that filled earlier stages of their lives.

That we all have such private internal struggles does not mean we are all frauds. Neither does the awareness of these painful emotions doom us to misery. These struggles mean simply that we all used to be vulnerable children, less capable of controlling our lives than we are now, and that a part of our brain will remember forever the vulnerability and fears that came with being young and small. As Harville Hendrix explains in *Getting the Love You Want: A Guide for Couples*,[7] these fears are stored in the *old brain* and very much shape both our personality and our reactions to one another.

The old brain consists of the most primitive portions of the brain, including the brain stem and the limbic system. Here, our minds are filled with hazy awarenesses of the external world, which stir automatic, self-protecting physical and psychological reactions. In contrast, the *new brain*—the cerebral cortex—is much more highly developed. Our new brain allows us to consciously choose reactions, to think and make decisions based on new information, and to plan and organize.

The reason our internal emotional struggles never seem to go away is that our old brain has no sense of time. Past, present, and future all blend together in this part of our mind. This is why we sometimes react to here-and-now stressors (for example, marital conflicts and heart illness) in ways that are alarmingly out of proportion to the events at hand. This is also why the psychological and behavioral ways we developed long ago to deal with life become rules for coping (deeply ingrained coping habits) that forever shape our reactions.

Because the primitive coping strategies that are stored in the old brain are the most familiar and automatic psychological reactions, they drive our behavior during stressful times. The higher the stress, the more driven we are to act in these old ways. Doing so feels necessary for emotional survival and just seems natural. Even if we know in our new brain that a different way of coping would work better, we automatically reach for the old, familiar reactions to soothe ourselves.

[7]H. Hendrix, *Getting the Love You Want: A Guide for Couples* (New York: Harper & Row, 1988).

After all, it is unlikely that we would further stress ourselves during scary, stressful times by trying new, unfamiliar ways of reacting.

The unfortunate truth is, however, that these most familiar ways of coping often backfire in our contemporary efforts to deal with life. These old-time coping patterns often fuel unhealthy ways of thinking and behaving—ways of coping that can work against both individual and marital health. As will be seen shortly, this is particularly true of coping with the stress of illness.

Nevertheless, personality change is not impossible. Even in reacting to something as stress generating as heart illness, we can learn new ways of coping. To do so, we must first accurately pinpoint our personality-based rules for coping. Then we must honestly determine if these overlearned ways of coping are actually interfering with our ability to make healthy choices in reacting to life stressors.

So what are *your* old-brain, personality-based rules for coping? What might be the negative health consequences of blindly following these rules to cope with heart illness? How do your personality patterns differ from your partner's? What effect does your personality have on your marital intimacy? And what can you do to update your old-brain rules and control your coping reactions?

There are many possible ways of discussing personality types and their behavioral consequences. However, this book is by no means intended to be about personality theory, so I have simplified the topic in the next section.

Personality Drivers

A practical and sensible perspective on personality and coping patterns is called transactional analysis.[8] This theory proposes, in part, that most of us can characterize our old-brain coping patterns as revolving around one or more of the following six themes. These patterns become so familiar and habitual that they seem to *drive* our perceptions, our behavioral choices, and our corresponding emotional

[8]I. Stewart and V. Joines, *TA Today: A New Introduction to Transactional Analysis* (Nottingham, England: Lifespace Publishing, 1987).

reactions in day-to-day living. These six *drivers* become especially influential in shaping our reactions during stressful times. As you read on, try to identify your own and your partner's most typical style of reacting to stress.

1. *Being Strong.* Individuals driven by this personality theme were taught to cope with life by being stoic and strong. Burdens are shouldered without complaint. Tasks are done without requests for help. Feelings of vulnerability and neediness are numbed or blocked from awareness. At the same time, selective attention is paid to "powerful" feelings, such as anger. When faced with life situations that overwhelm them with feelings of fear and need for help, such people experience shame and discomfort. These uncomfortable feelings of vulnerability interfere with the Being Strong person's ability to ask for openly or to accept graciously emotional support from others.

2. *Being Perfect.* Anxiety and guilt fill the lives of people who are stuck in efforts to be perfect, because perfection is never attained. But the old brain of a Being Perfect personality does not know this, and it is as though such people have been taught that if they can just "do it perfectly," then their internal anxiety will go away. The "it" can be anything: cleaning the house, exercising, getting information about one's medical condition, or straightening pictures on a wall. Living life this way creates a gut-wrenching trap: the less perfect the outcomes, the more guilt and anxiety drive renewed efforts to quiet the pain by further pursuing perfection.

3. *Trying Hard.* These people have learned to feel valued for their ability to try harder than the next guy. It is as though their self-worth is based on fatiguing themselves by struggling longer and harder than others. Life is seen as filled with tasks and obligations. Trying Hard personalities have difficulty determining when they have worked hard enough to deserve a rest. They feel anxious if they try to relax or play. The more anxious they feel, the harder they work, often to a degree that proves detrimental to their own well-being.

4. *Pleasing Others.* These people live as though they had been put on earth to take care of others. They have difficulty being appropriately self-focused and self-nurturing without feeling guilt. They therefore have much difficulty with setting appropriate limits for responding to the needs of others and giving clear expression to their own

needs. Indeed, such people have trouble identifying their internal needs accurately. They often give to others the kind of attention and nurturance they would like to receive, but they have difficulty asking directly for gifts of love and attention.

Because they do not take appropriate care of themselves within relationships, Pleasing Others personalities often end up feeling drained and martyred by others. Periods of exhausted withdrawal (perhaps into depression) often result. But the old brain then kicks in with guilt- and fear-generating messages that Pleasing Others is the safest way to be. Then the old patterns of self-sacrificing caretaking return.

5. *Hurrying.* Some of us do not know how to feel comfortable with a reasonably paced life-style because we have always been taught to rush. Throughout childhood many of us were told repeatedly to hurry up, usually by parents who were overstressed by busy schedules. The Hurrying message continues in adulthood as we fill our lives with more to do than time allows. It is therefore understandable that an old-brain message driving many people is that hurrying is necessary to survive. People who are driven by a Hurrying message grow accustomed to an internal sense of urgency. They experience uncomfortable frustration, agitation, and anxiety if forced to slow down.

6. *Being Careful.* Some people learn that living is a frightening proposition at best. Constant old-brain warnings about being careful stir free-floating anxieties (fears that are not attached to any specific stimulus). Being Careful people particularly experience obsessive worrying and distressing anxiety in reaction to life changes, big or small. They are therefore likely to monitor their own and others' reactions excessively during times of transition. This is because they have learned to doubt their own or others' abilities to cope with the consequences of events that change the status quo. Because they are constantly on guard, Being Careful people have difficulty relaxing and enjoying themselves. Their anxieties can grow to interfere with most aspects of their life.

Most of us can identify with parts of each of these coping patterns. Indeed, each of these ways of being is an appropriate and adaptive response to some life situations some of the time. The problem is that our old brain does not tell us when it is safe *not* to use these coping strategies. We all get stuck sometimes in extreme versions of these patterns and have difficulty trusting the intellectual message coming from our new brain, telling us it is safe to try an alternative coping strategy that is more appropriate. Our fear and discomfort with the unfamiliar propel us back into the already overused coping strategies. In this way, our very efforts to cope become a source of—not a solution to—our stress. The driver that got us here leads us still deeper into pain-filled territory. The story of Carly and George demonstrates this process.

Carly had spent her life caring for others. As the oldest of three children, she was her mother's helpmate throughout her childhood, cooking, cleaning, baby-sitting, and generally learning to attend to the needs of others as a means of earning looks of approval and words of praise. She eventually became so stuck in this way of reacting that she felt comfortable only when she was taking care of others, even if she received no words of appreciation.

Marrying George and mothering their three children continued Carly's life pattern of Pleasing Others. Her husband's long work hours and driving ambition left Carly exclusively in charge of nurturing her loved ones. This was a role for which she was naturally suited and in which she had always thrived.

And then George had a heart attack. This event led to Carly's facing a very unfamiliar and unsettling dilemma. At first, things went on comfortably as usual. Carly was certainly comfortable in the role of caretaker; George's new status as heart patient in need of care fit nicely with Carly's Pleasing Others personality. However, as the fears and stresses of George's recuperation evolved from the event of hospitalization to the multiple dramas throughout his first year of recovery, Carly found herself privately overwhelmed with fatigue, depression, and—most confusing to her—anger toward George.

Her nurturing tone of attending to George by reminding him to take his medication, eat sensibly, and to work less gradually shifted into a more bitter-sounding refrain. To her horror, George began complaining about her constant nagging, and he even accused her of not being supportive or understanding of his struggle to cope with his illness.

In reaction to George's feedback, Carly felt depressing guilt. She convinced herself that George was correct; she had become self-centered in her discontent. After all, she wasn't the one who had gone through the terror of having a heart attack. She redoubled her commitment to being more helpful to George. She went through the nurturing motions. She was plagued by a painful sadness, however. She kept quiet about this pain; no sense "nagging" any more.

Within months, Carly was having migraine headaches regularly. Her own doctor urged her to take better care of herself, to take time for relaxation and pleasure in her life, and to let her emotional needs be known more clearly. In line with her Pleasing Others personality, Carly tried to please her doctor and follow his advice. She declared one night a week Mom's night off for eating out with the family and taking a break from cooking. She rejoined her neighborhood walking group, which she had dropped after George's heart attack. She even went to a few movies with friends as a special treat to herself.

The problem was that whenever Carly tried to nurture herself in these sensible and reasonable ways, she felt more discomfort than relief. In fact, the guilt and anxiety she felt while trying to enjoy any break from her caretaker role was so intense that it overrode the potential pleasure. She experienced moments of internal calming only when she returned to some activity that involved caring for George or their children. Such excessive caretaking might be exhausting and depressing and ultimately stress her into having migraines, but at least she felt as if she was doing what she was "supposed" to be doing to be a worthwhile person.

George's story parallels Carly's, but it revolves around a different personality theme. George was the third of six children in a financially poor family. His childhood was filled with hard work and the emotional pain of being physically smaller than his peers. In reaction, George learned that a combination of Being Strong and Trying Hard was the best way to soothe his internal fears. His life became an endless quest to rise above his upbringing by being strong enough to work harder than the next guy in whatever he undertook.

When he married Carly, he did so with an unspoken vow to provide a more comfortable life for her and their eventual family than he had experienced as a child. This commitment translated into working long hours in his profession as an accountant for a large corporation. His annual performance evaluations consistently rewarded him for his diligence and obvious commitment to the company. Such praise, and its accompanying financial rewards, further fueled George's quest. He worked longer and harder than his peers. He denied awareness of fatigue and refused to miss work for minor illnesses, despite Carly's warnings that he was working himself into poor health. George constantly motivated himself with the belief that he was getting progressively closer to the day when he and his loving family would relax and enjoy life, safe and secure beneath the protective umbrella of the success that he had finally achieved.

And then he had his heart attack. George's life came to a screeching halt, but his emotional sense of urgency speeded up. He endured the initial months of posthospitalization rehabilitation without complaint but with a growing restlessness to return to work. He feared that the promotion he had worked so hard for would never materialize unless he fully and immediately recovered from this illness. He approached each day as another opportunity to prove his recovery by denying, even to himself, the existence of any fears, symptoms, or lingering effects of his heart condition.

Carly's helpful encouragement and nurturing meant more to George throughout these months than he told her. After all, if he admitted that he was benefiting from such reassurance, he might imply that he needed it. He feared for the effects of his illness on his wife and his children, and he assumed that the best way to reassure them would be to demonstrate a speedy and problem-free return to work.

Even though he did soon return to work full-time, George was haunted by a confusing feeling of emptiness. As he had done throughout his life, he tried to distract himself from his inner pain by working harder, achieving more, and getting busier. But he seemed to be on an emotional treadmill. The harder he worked in stoic disregard of his feelings of vulnerability, the uneasier he felt. The uneasier he felt, the harder he worked, and so on.

As George's tension and fatigue mounted, he became more irritable with Carly, with their children, and with life in general. When Carly began experiencing migraine headaches he seethed with guilt and self-loathing; he assumed that her problems were due to the stress that his illness and long working hours had created. To soothe his wife, George proclaimed his intention to work less and begin smelling the roses more. For six weeks he tore himself away from work in time to be home for dinner with the family. On weekends he resisted his pre-occupying agitation to go in to the office. But even though he was there in body, his time spent at home was far less than emotionally satisfying. Carly looked depressed. He and she seemed to be relating superficially rather than intimately. Work was piling up at the office. He began to have difficulty sleeping through the night because he tossed and turned, worrying about unfinished work details and about his growing problems at home.

When the year-end busy season finally arrived at George's company, the pressure to return to his old ways was too much to resist. Gradually, George once again began to work late on weekdays and to return to the office on weekends. His familiar internal numbness returned, and his wife seemed more distant than ever. But now at least he could sleep at night.

The Hard Work of Psychological Change

It is obvious that both George and Carly were aware of the behavioral changes they needed to make for more appropriate and comfortable balance in their lives. Carly tried to move from blindly following her Pleasing Others driver by taking time for self-nurturing activities. George tried to counter his Being Strong and Trying Hard drivers by working less and by spending more time with his family. But these positive changes did not immediately help these well-intentioned people.

The experiences of Carly and George demonstrate three important psychological facts:

1. Changing old coping patterns does not feel good at first. Healthy psychological changes often stir feelings of awkwardness or fears that we are making a mistake in behaving this new way.

2. To truly change in healthy ways, we must put up with the anxiety until the new way of operating becomes more familiar. The initial anxiety does not mean we are making a mistake; it simply signals that we are in unfamiliar territory.

3. The longer we explore the new territory, the more familiar and comfortable it will become.

We need nurturing support and encouragement from each other as we grapple with the anxieties that are provoked when new psychological territory is being explored. Unfortunately, far too many couples get caught in the trap of struggling with solo attempts to change. Such couples, like Carly and George, grow more and more lonely within the privacy of their own marriage.

How you can be sources of healing for each other is extensively discussed in later chapters. Here I simply want to emphasize that it is important and helpful to be aware of each other's personality-based coping tendencies, and to be open in asking for and offering each other support and encouragement as you each strive to develop healthier ways of dealing with life.

In helping each other to cope more positively with the unique stresses of illness, it is useful to understand the coping consequences of the various personality drivers. It is to this topic that we now turn.

Why Do We Act This Way?

In my work as a psychotherapist and marital therapist, I have noticed that each of the driver coping patterns leads us into predictable areas of distress if used excessively in efforts to cope with change. Furthermore, I have found that the different kinds of distress that correspond with the different drivers lead to certain problems in reacting to illness. By understanding these potential personality-based pitfalls in coping with illness, you can avoid much pain and confusion. To help each other, you must understand what both of you are trying to accomplish—accomplish psychologically, that is—by behaving as you do.

Certain well-intentioned, healthy hopes and needs underlie most of our coping strategies. This makes common sense; we cope in ways we hope will allow us to end a negative state of affairs, gain a positive outcome, or avoid a feared negative outcome. It often seems that we operate as though we believe that if we can just do or be _____ (our typical coping pattern) long enough and hard enough, then _____ (the corresponding hoped-for, soothing consequence) will finally occur. A double-crossing surprise for most of us, however, is that the harder we do or be _____ (that is, follow our driver), the more thoroughly we stay stuck in an unanticipated pit of distress.

The underlying hopes that typically correspond with each of the major coping patterns are outlined in table 9.1. This table also outlines the pitfalls that inevitably result from excessively following any given driver in coping with stress. I recommend that you and your spouse review table 9.1 together. Identify any symptoms that might describe your reactions as you fall prey to coping pitfalls. Note the underlying hopes that probably correspond with your misguided efforts to deal with stress by overusing your particular drivers.

Certainly no one (not even a concerned spouse) can change for you, but you can be helpful to each other as you attempt to change yourselves. It will be tremendously soothing if you will bless each other by providing some version of the hopes that underlie the driver

Table 9.1 Coping Patterns and Pitfalls

Driver	Underlying Hope	Coping Pitfalls
Being Strong	To be nurtured	Numbness, loneliness, anger
Being Perfect	To feel good enough	Guilt, anxiety, obsessive preoccupation, aloofness
Trying Hard	To feel deserving of rest and enjoyment	Exhaustion, stress, depression, joylessness
Pleasing Others	To feel understood and appreciated	Exhaustion, withdrawal, guilt
Hurrying	To feel finished	Frazzled and chaotic feelings
Being Careful	To feel safe	Free-floating fear and obsessive worrying

patterns as each of you attempts your respective changing. For example, it is helpful to a Trying Hard individual to be reminded by his or her spouse that he or she deserves to rest and enjoy life. Or, in countering Being Perfect tendencies, it is helpful to be reminded that "good enough" is all that is required in most aspects of life.

After reviewing and discussing table 9.1, list the coping patterns each of you wants to modify. Next, list the ways you can be nurturingly helpful to each other as you struggle with the anxieties of learning about these new ways of being.

The Personality Drivers and Heart Illness

Any personality is capable of making unhealthy choices in reacting to the stress of illness. In table 9.2, the various unhealthy reactions to illness that often correspond with each of the major coping patterns are listed. By understanding these potential problems in dealing with the stress of illness, you can avoid or correct much marital turmoil.

Again, I recommend that the two of you read this table and the following explanations together. Identify your own and each other's coping patterns in reacting to illness. Use this information to help each other begin more open and flexible ways of dealing with the impact that this illness has had on your marriage.

Being Strong in hopes of eventually being nurtured requires that you remain numb to your own feelings. Irritability, anger, and an overall feeling of being alone in one's struggle are the inevitable results of this mode of coping with illness. For some, depression follows. Because the Being Strong personality does not directly ask for support, other family members may eventually stop offering support, no matter how concerned they are. Family tensions then mount as the Being Strong individual begins to feel unnurtured, particularly by the spouse.

Such people lose sight of the fact that they are not letting their needs be known; they think anyone who loves them ought to *know* that they feel vulnerable beneath the outer layers of coping strength.

If the heart patient follows a Being Strong coping pattern, seeming or actual denial of the medical realities of his or her condition often

Table 9.2 Coping Patterns and Reactions to Illness

Driver	Maladaptive Reaction to Illness
Being Strong	Quiet about one's own fears and needs; seeming denial of all concerns; eventual depression from perception that others do not care; focus on physical symptoms as indirect way to get soothed.
Being Perfect	Obsessiveness about details of health; all-or-nothing thinking; ignoring the spirit of the rehabilitation process; never soothed that adherence to details of rehabilitation is sufficient.
Trying Hard	Sense of urgency that interferes with pacing; attitude of "wait until" rehabilitation is completed before enjoying life.
Pleasing Others	Lack of self-expression; failure to soothe own needs; guilt over illness that interferes with needed relief from performing "well enough"; fear; discomfort telling medical personnel anything that might disappoint them.
Hurrying	Frustration, irritability, and impatience with slowness of own or others' progress in recovering or adapting; demoralized; resort to "quick cures."
Being Careful	Fear-based withdrawal from life; spectatoring; obsessive monitoring of own or others' reactions; depression.

occurs. Some of these folks simply block out awareness of physical symptoms such as chest pain or shortness of breath and thereby fail to make needed adjustments in their activity levels. Others deny the very existence of heart disease, something that is relatively easy to do given its invisibility.

I periodically see Being Strong patients who are denying their illness with such statements as, "My doctors and my spouse claim I had a heart attack, but I believe all I had was a bad case of indigestion." Of course, such denial is quite frightening to concerned family members. Fear that an ill spouse is not taking heart disease seriously often leads families to develop stress-generating patterns of monitoring the patient's behavior. Having one's behavior monitored is quite uncomfortable for a person who is accustomed to Being Strong and independent, and a spiraling of relationship tensions often results.

Although Being Strong typically involves not directly asking for attention, help, or nurturing from others—certainly a lonely way to live—I have noticed that some Being Strong people develop a different and somewhat surprising coping pattern that contrasts with the denial shown by many Being Strong heart patients: they become excessively focused on physical symptoms. They overattend to physical ailments, suggesting that they derive some form of emotional gain from remaining in a sick role. I am convinced that some Being Strong personalities do indeed become uniquely soothed and nurtured in reaction to illness behavior. Such people are certainly *not* faking it. The increased love and attention that often come from others when one is sick can lead to such relief from loneliness that the sick behavior becomes unconsciously exaggerated. In this way, the Being Strong heart patient avoids returning to living in emotional isolation.

Of course, these Being Strong patterns do not apply only to heart patients. A spouse, too, can get stuck in Being Strong in trying to be a source of stability for a sick mate. The potential costs of this pattern are similar for spouses and patients: feelings of aloneness and depression, physical symptoms that become aggravated by the stress of the caretaker role, quiet resentments toward the sick partner, and general exhaustion from caretaker burnout.

Personalities driven by *Being Perfect* have trouble feeling satisfied with their own performance in life. Guilt, anxiety, and obsessive preoccupation with the flaws of their lives often lead such persons to appear aloof and critical. They may seem stuck in the habit of criticizing others, but the truth is that their own internal self-criticism is their greatest enemy.

Trying to be perfect in coping with heart illness leads to predictable problems. Such people tend to (1) worry obsessively about the details of illness and the rehabilitation process or (2) develop rigid and ritualistic rehabilitation routines. Such reactions to illness inevitably prove irritating to others. Any spouse grows tired of dealing with someone who is never satisfied with "good enough" progress, or who refuses to participate in even a reasonable degree of spontaneous changing of daily routines. A heart patient or a spouse driven by attempts at Being Perfect tends to drive the other person crazy with aggravation.

The great double-cross in the lives of people who are driven by *Trying Hard* personality scripts is that they feel deserving of rest and enjoyment only if they are exhausted from excessive work and worry. Of course, not much pleasure is possible when you are exhausted, so Trying Hard personalities seldom have much fun. Rather, they tend to stress themselves into chronic, mild levels of depression of the sort that results from working too hard at being a hard worker.

This excessive work ethic interferes with the Trying Hard individual's ability to be comfortable with a reasonably paced rehabilitation process. An inner sense of urgency propels these people to expect and demand an accelerated rehabilitation course. Such people also tend to put enjoyment of life on hold until the rehabilitation is over with. They make the mistake of conceptualizing cardiac rehabilitation as an event that can be shortened by extra effort. One such individual verbalized this attitude in reaction to her husband's participation in a cardiac rehabilitation program this way: "We figure our lives will get back to normal once my husband's rehab is done. Everything is on hold until then. If this program is based on exercising three times a week, wouldn't he cut his rehabilitation period in half if he exercised six times a week?"

The truth, of course, is that cardiac rehabilitation is a lifelong process, and not an event with a clear beginning middle, and end. The urgent and impatient spirit of the Trying Hard individual often leads to poor rehabilitation choices, such as exercising excessively or adopting unrealistic expectations about how quickly rehabilitation goals will be met. Such excessive Trying Hard typically leads to feelings of being demoralized and frustrated, both with oneself and with others. These feelings interfere with maintaining supportive, encouraging relationships of the sort that are necessary for the Trying Hard personality to learn a new coping pattern in reaction to illness.

Pleasing Others personalities become anxious when they perceive others as being in need of help, support, or understanding. They give excessive nurturing to others for two reasons: (1) To do so feels natural and personally gratifying; and (2) they have an underlying hope that caring for others will lead to their being appreciated and nurtured in return. This way of living often leads to exhaustion and periods of withdrawal; shouldering the emotional needs of others can wear you out. Most of us have no trouble giving ourselves permission to take a break from being a caretaker occasionally, but Pleasing Others personalities may experience extreme guilt and anxiety if they actually do say no to others.

This coping pattern can result in various unhealthy reactions to illness. For example, because they do not clearly express their own emotional needs, Pleasing Others personalities may go through the rehabilitation process filled with feelings of loneliness. This difficulty with self-expression even leads some such people to remain quiet about medical concerns when visiting their physicians. As one person explained, "My cardiologist is the most caring man! I can see how badly he wants me to get well. I just hate to disappoint him by complaining about my chest pains."

Pleasing Others personalities also blame themselves excessively for any discomfort they cause others. Guilt is an inevitable consequence. In this vein, heart patients may blame themselves for putting their families "through all this." In parallel, Pleasing Others family members may blame themselves "for not having done something to prevent this illness from happening." The guilt is never quite soothed, regardless of how hard such people work to please others. Because of their constant guilt, they never feel quite satisfied with rehabilitation efforts, their own or their partner's.

Hurrying personalities are similar to Trying Hard copers in their sense of urgency about completing the tasks that face them. However, these people typically feel frazzled and chaotic in response to their urgency, versus the sense of steadfast goal-directedness experienced by Trying Hard personalities.

Hurrying personalities experience much frustration and irritability when faced with the reality that cardiac rehabilitation is a lifelong process, not an event that will soon be finished. They may become impatient and critical in their dealings with others. This just creates even more tension, which further fuels their frustration with the slow pace of rehabilitation. This frustration can escalate into loss of motivation to continue reasonable and sensible rehabilitation efforts. Two poor choices made by some who are caught in the Hurrying trap are (1) foolishly attempting dangerous quick cure methods and (2) completely giving up out of impatience and frustration with the rehabilitation process.

Steven was a case in point. He had always lived in a frantic rush. He often appeared disorganized and overwhelmed as he rushed about, usually expressing an urgent need to hurry because he was running late for his next appointment. After many years of struggling to control his chronically high blood pressure, Steven suffered a serious myocardial infarction. He was also forty-five pounds over ideal body weight. His comments about needing to lose weight typify the dangerous coping trap experienced by Hurrying cardiac patients:

"First, my doctor told me to start exercising a few times a week, so I did. Then he told me to eat less junk food, so I did. I dropped ten pounds during the first two weeks, but I haven't lost any more weight in the past three months. Now he's telling me I have to lose fifty pounds or this blood pressure treatment won't work. And he's saying I should only lose one or two pounds a week or the weight won't stay off.

"Give me a break! At two pounds a week, it would take twenty-five weeks to lose this weight. At one pound a week, it would take almost a year! I've never done anything consistently for an entire year in my life. If there's not a quicker way to do this, then I'm not doing it. Maybe I'll just fast for a month, or just drink juices or something. If that doesn't work, then I don't know, maybe I'll just take my chances being fat."

Remember that if either of you becomes trapped in Hurrying patterns you run the risk of damaging both your marital harmony and the cardiac rehabilitation progress. Coping with any chronic illness requires patience and the ability to accept that progress may sometimes go slowly—virtues that are difficult for Hurrying personalities to grasp.

If *Being Careful* is the main personality driver, then life becomes an endless attempt to worry enough to feel safe. Of course, because worrying and feeling safe do not mix well, this hoped-for peace of mind is never attained.

Following a Being Careful script in coping with illness leads to obsessive monitoring of everyone's reactions. Such people can be described as living out a spectatoring role in life; they observe and worry, rather than participate in and enjoy each day. The result is significant lessening of marital and family intimacy levels. Being Careful spectators not only are anguished by internal worries, but also create anguish in relationships with their worrying, warning, and whining.

Being Careful copers also tend to become depressed because their worrying keeps them from participating in the mainstream of life; they withdraw from the roles that typically define and determine their life's meaning. They then begin to question their own worth and value as their self-esteem suffers. Such depressing withdrawal from life works against rehabilitation from illness. Improving quality of life, not withdrawing from life, should be the motivating cornerstone of successful cardiac rehabilitation.

Summary

This overview is far from a complete synopsis of personality theory, but it should suffice to make several important points. First, it is obvious that *psychological reactions to illness are varied and often complex.* I trust, however, that I have clearly conveyed my sincere belief that, second, *psychological change and healthy control of coping patterns are possible in coping with illness.* Such positive adjusting is hard and sometimes confusing work, but it is work that each of us can do, with each other's help.

Third, helping each other to cope healthily with illness requires (1) a basic understanding of each other's coping patterns, (2) the courage to steer your own reactions in healthy directions, (3) the perseverance to put up with discomfort until new coping patterns begin to feel familiar, and (4) loving support of each other while you both are learning new ways of reacting.

The preceding pages can serve as helpful guidelines to you and your family in identifying the areas where emotional support is most needed as well as the riskiest pitfalls in the process of adjusting to illness. Read them and reread them. Discuss your reactions with each other. Pay particular attention to the descriptions that strike you as on target about your own or each other's styles of coping, and check your impressions with each other. Such honest self-appraisal and open discussion might be uncomfortable at first, but remember that *positive psychological change most often feels awkward until this new way of being becomes more familiar.*

When all goes well with partners who are trying to cope with illness, they become more tender, patient, compassionate, and relaxed as they celebrate the goodness of their life together. Unfortunately, these psychological characteristics are contrary to those that exist at the foundation level of a unique breed of personality so often seen in cardiac rehabilitation settings: the Type A personality. Living with a Type A personality and being a Type A personality pose special tasks in the process of establishing and maintaining intimate connections. We now turn to a discussion of the dilemmas facing couples that organize around the Type A behavior pattern.

Ten

Marriage and
Type A Personalities

∎ ∎ ∎ ∎ ∎

One of the contributions of cardiac rehabilitation and cardiac research has been the identification of the Type A personality. If poorly controlled, this unique breed of coping can increase the risk of developing heart illness and decrease the odds of recovering from heart disease.

Cardiologists Meyer Friedman and Ray Rosenman originated the concept of the Type A behavior pattern from their observations of their patient population. Friedman and Rosenman originally defined this behavior pattern as "an action-emotion complex that can be observed in any person who is aggressively involved in a chronic incessant struggle to achieve more and more in less and less time, and if required to do so, against the opposing efforts of other things or other persons."[9]

These are tense, energetic individuals who live as if driven by some inner boiler of energy. They approach life with a sense of competitive aggressiveness. They are often referred to as "workaholics." They seem to suffer from "hurry sickness" in that they tend to do everything in a quick and urgent manner.

Type A's can be quite controlling in relationships. They operate as

[9]M. Friedman and R. Rosenman, *Type A Behavior and Your Heart* (New York: Alfred A. Knopf, 1974), p. 67.

160

though their way of doing things is the only correct course to follow. Their personal power—coupled with a sometimes quick temper, often explosive speech, and typically tense facial musculature—can be quite intimidating. Their typical style is to think and do more than one thing at a time. As a result, they often give the impression of not paying full attention during conversation. Type A's tend to interrupt when others are speaking and to break eye contact because of distracting thoughts or distracting reactions to environmental stimuli.

These people may also show excessive anger and irritation when faced with any frustrating obstacle. Both large and small hassles can lead to these angry reactions. For Type A's, being unable to find a needed ingredient while preparing a meal could be just as infuriating as being interrupted unnecessarily during an important business meeting. For some, these anger reactions become so pervasive that the individuals appear to be driven by generalized hostility.

Type A behavior pattern has historically been observed primarily in men, but contemporary women are rapidly catching up. Type A women appear as a variation on this coping theme. Perhaps because women are traditionally socialized not to express anger openly, many Type A females show a different set of symptoms: generalized frustration, irritation, and depression. Rather than openly display hostility (like male Type A's), female Type A's are more likely to suffer the signs of holding back powerful emotions. Teeth grinding, exhaustion, and a general sense of drivenness to be all things to all people are frequently seen in Type A women. These are people who quietly push themselves with perfectionistic self-standards in all that they do.

I do not mean to imply that every ambitious, energetic, hard-working person is a Type A personality, or that everyone who is a Type A personality will develop heart disease. Many such hard drivers are exceptionally happy and healthy. The hallmark characteristic of the problem Type A behavior pattern, however, is joylessness. Extreme Type A's are said to be locked into a joyless striving for accomplishment.

This is not to say that Type A's never smile; it simply means that they are seldom truly satisfied with themselves or others for any length of time, because they are predisposed to respond in a Type A manner to situations they perceive as challenges to their need for control. The problem is that Type A's tend to perceive *most* aspects of life as challenges and therefore tend to wear out themselves and others with their time urgency, perfectionism, competitiveness, and hostility as they struggle to maintain control of themselves and of the people and situations that they encounter.

Nor do I mean to imply that any individual who has heart disease is a Type A personality. Many of my heart patients are so-called Type B personalities—those who have a relaxed, unhurried, gracious, non-competitive style of responding. Some people evidence a combination of Type A and Type B personality characteristics. When a Type B patient has a Type A spouse, then the spouse, not the patient, may react to heart illness in a Type A flurry. For such patients, dealing with the spouse's Type A reactions to cardiac rehabilitation can be the most difficult part of recovery.

How familiar do these descriptions sound to you? Is this familiarity based on what you see of yourself or on your experiences in living with your spouse? As you answer, remember that no one is an *absolute* Type A; not all aspects of this syndrome need be present for an individual to be considered Type A. Many of us evidence some Type A characteristic (for example, hurry sickness) in one setting (for example, at work), but not in others (for example, at home). Others consistently show some, but not all, of the Type A responses, regardless of the situation. Such a person, for example, may generally react with quiet competitiveness, perfectionism, and hostility—both at work and at home—but may not typically interact with others in a manner that is openly hostile.

It is important to be honest about whether you are stuck in Type A ways of reacting. Based both on my extensive review of many of the more than two thousand professional publications regarding the Type A behavior pattern and on my own clinical experience, I am certain that *extreme, unchecked Type A reactivity on the part of either marriage partner significantly interferes with the cardiac rehabilitation process and universally disrupts marital and family intimacy.*

Please read that statement again, and note two important points. First, I emphasize that the deterrent to rehabilitation for Type A's is "extreme, unchecked" reactivity. Recent research has suggested that

Type A heart patients who learn to modify their typical styles of reactivity rehabilitate from heart illness more successfully than Type A's who do not modify their behavior and that these reformed Type A's may even be more successful in accomplishing cardiac rehabilitation than their Type B counterparts.

What does this mean? It means the Type A style is not necessarily deadly, but extreme Type A reactivity certainly is dangerous.

Second, I emphasize my impression that any extreme Type A reactivity within a marital team—whether that Type A-ness is shown by the heart patient or by the spouse—is detrimental both to the marriage and to the rehabilitation process. Such behavior works against the creation of emotional support and intimacy of the sort that is necessary for effective marital and family functioning and that enhances cardiac rehabilitation. Let me put it in other words:

Marital and family intimacy enhances cardiac rehabilitation.

Marital and family stress works against cardiac rehabilitation.

Extreme Type A behavior interferes with marital and family intimacy.

Therefore, extreme Type A behavior is bad for heart patients and for families.

The impact of Type A behavior pattern on marriages is a relatively unresearched area (a peculiar and unfortunate fact). I am convinced that the greatest and most accurate source of information about the inner workings of Type A personalities is not cardiologists or psychologists or psychiatrists or physiological researchers. The inexhaustible (and relatively untapped) fount of information about these driven people is the people who live with them.

Spouses see beyond the Type A's intimidating bravado. Family members grow to understand the often sensitive and brittle cores of such personalities. But these same family members are also the most frequent targets (victims?) of the Type A person's style of reacting.

In keeping with the theme of this book, the following pages explore the topic of how to manage the cardiac risk factor of Type A behavior pattern from a marital perspective. (This chapter could be called "How to be married to a Type A and live to tell about it.") As you read on, remember that these descriptions probably apply, to some degree, to one or both of you. No one exhibits all these characteristics, and everyone exhibits some of them.

The important point is not to label your partner or yourself in some categorizing way. The important point is to learn to recognize and modify any Type A coping patterns that may be generating distress in your relationship or for you as individuals and that may therefore be interfering with cardiac rehabilitation.

In exploring this topic, I first give a brief overview of specific factors that are helpful in understanding the Type A individual and that should be addressed by anyone trying to change Type A patterns. I then discuss the underlying psychological and physiological causes and operations of Type A responsivity. Finally, I discuss the impact of Type A-ness on marital and family life.

How to Tell Who Is Type A

There are no absolute personality types. Every individual is unique, and all of us are simply doing the best we can to cope, on the basis of what we have learned from our past experiences. Bearing this in mind, it is most helpful to think of Type A-ness as a set of habitual responses that result from an interaction between personal and environmental factors. As was already stated, this style of coping is typically most blatant when Type A individuals are actively responding to things that are important to them, or when they are challenged or frustrated in their efforts. At such times, Type A behavior follows fairly predictable paths related to a variety of factors.

What characteristics distinguish the Type A style of coping? This question has been addressed in literally thousands of research studies. Noteworthy in this realm of research are the works of C. David Jenkins, Virginia Price, Redford Williams, and Meyer Friedman with Ray Rosenman and Diane Ulmer.[10] The summary of the Type A re-

[10]C.D. Jenkins, Psychologic and social precursors of coronary disease, *New England Journal of Medicine* 284 (1971): 244–55. V. Price, *Type A Behavior Pattern: A Model for Research and Practice* (New York: Academic Press, 1982). R. Williams, *The Trusting Heart: Great News about Type A Behavior* (New York: Time Books, 1989). M. Friedman and

sponse style in table 10.1 is based on my review of this literature and on my extensive work with hundreds of Type A men and women. Let me again emphasize that no single person manifests every characteristic listed in the table. It is also true that every Type B person occasionally displays some of these same characteristics.

In determining the extent of your Type A reactivity, it is helpful to note the severity of your responses in different situations. Do you react alike to both minor and major stressors? Are you able to calm your reactions quickly, or do you end up feeling out of control of your reactions? Extreme Type A's are like furnaces with faulty thermostats; they do the job of altering the environment, but they never pause or regulate their effort. They seem to be stuck on a high setting of reactivity. The result is a constant expenditure of energy, premature aging of the "machine" (the body), and notable discomfort for everyone in the affected environment.

A number of contemporary researchers have emphasized that not all aspects of the Type A style of reacting are equally toxic with regard to causing heart disease. Convincingly summarizing his own and others' research, Redford Williams of Duke University Medical Center emphasized the toxicity of three components of Type A reactivity: cynical mistrust of others, which leads to frequently experiencing anger, which in turn results in frequent, overt expression of hostility to others.[11]

Individuals caught in this cycle of habitual hostile response to the world are thought to be at highest risk of developing coronary artery disease. It also seems quite likely to me that family members who are the targets of a Type A caught in this cynicism-anger-hostility triad are also at significant risk—of being miserable.

A logical question at this juncture might be, "Why in the world would anyone want to be and behave this way?" (If you are truly Type A, an equally normal question for you to ask right now might be, "Why doesn't this 'expert' just get on with it? I don't have time to

---

R. Rosenman, *Type A Behavior and Your Heart* (New York: Alfred A. Knopf, 1974). M. Friedman and D. Ulmer, *Treating Type A Behavior and Your Heart* (New York: Alfred A. Knopf, 1984).

[11]R. Williams, *The Trusting Heart*, p. 44–71.

Table 10.1 **Summary of Type A Response Styles**

Values

Conscientious and responsible in an inflexible way.

Driven by perfectionism, which is expected of self and of others.

Evaluates own and others' goodness and worth based on productivity rather than on any other qualities, or just on being.

Craves recognition and power.

Attracted compulsively to the competition and challenge aspects of an activity to a degree that interferes with enjoying a game or activity with self or other, even with one's own children.

Derives gratification primarily from work and from leadership roles and therefore does not value activities that are purely relaxing and enjoyable in a passive way.

Mistrusts others.

Has a generally negative view of humanity that involves seeing others as unworthy, deceptive, and selfish.

Style of thinking

Tends to think and behave on several levels at once (works while eating, reads during a conversation, dictates while driving).

Constantly anticipates what is coming next and begins to react in advance (interrupts with answer before question is completed; gets keys out long before getting to the door; while driving, gets into turn lane long before coming to the turning point).

Hypervigilant: constantly scans surroundings, often noticing things that irritate (for example, someone in the grocery store express checkout line with eleven items in the basket instead of the clearly posted limit of ten).

Overaware of time as a factor: constantly struggles with the perception that there is not enough time to do all the things that he or she deems to be important and strives to do perfectly.

Poor observer of surroundings or of own behavior or own impact of others.

Interpersonal relationships

Self-centered.

Poor listener: gives many anticipatory nods and "ahems" and short explosive laughs in anticipation of the speaker's comments.

Easily bored by anyone different from self.

Table 10.1 Continued

Easily angered (sometimes seems to have hostility looking for a place to happen): honks horn at others while driving, glares at waiters for poor performance, reacts critically rather than nurturingly to others' mistakes.

Denies hostile feelings and disagrees with feedback given by others who observe hostile reactions.

Often frustrated when working closely with others.

Expresses overt bravado and certainty of own correctness and superior abilities.

Controlling: gives unsolicited advice and criticism.

Appears to be uncomfortable with physical intimacy or with verbal expressions of tender feelings.

Behaviors

Tense, energetic: often clenches hands or makes fists.

Explosively emphasizes points during conversation by pounding table or pointing finger in a parental manner.

Violently expresses opinions, using such words as "stupid," "ridiculous," "irresponsible," and "idiotic" in response to opinions differing from own.

Frequently uses profanity.

In perpetual motion: fidgets, taps feet, drums knuckles, shakes leg or foot.

Flashes tense smiles that look more like grimaces than indications of pleasurable reactions.

Tenses jaw muscles when emphasizing comments, resulting in a clipped speaking pattern.

Breathes irregularly, often resulting in expiratory sighs in the midst of conversations.

Constantly rushing, in a hurry, fighting against time constraints.

Hyperaggressive: tries to dominate, not just win, in a perceived competition, even at the expense of the other person's self-esteem.

waste reading all this descriptive garbage. These psychology types explain everything until they bore you to death.")

In getting answers to either of these questions, it is helpful to understand the physical and psychological factors that are thought to contribute to the Type A behavior pattern.

Causes and Core-Level Issues

No universally accepted explanation of the causes of any human behavior pattern exists. Any topic that receives a large amount of behavioral, psychological, and medical research attention generates a fair
amount of controversy, and this is certainly true for Type A reactivity.
Human behavior is simply too complex to be summed up in definitive
statements about what causes us to act the way we do.

Although human behavior is too complex to be neatly packaged
once and for all, much information does exist that can help you better
understand and manage the effect of the Type A pattern on your marriage. The observations of spouses of Type A's, plus the psychological
and medical facts that are summarized in this chapter, shed considerable light on the inner workings of Type A personalities.

Confessions of Spouses of Type A's

I believe that spouses of Type A individuals are invaluable sources of
information about these complex people. Many of my counseling
hours are spent with wives and husbands of Type A's, from whom I
have learned to appreciate that most Type A's are walking paradoxes:
powerful yet insecure; demanding yet sometimes quite generous and
self-sacrificing; multitalented yet seemingly unable to change certain
behaviors that they realize are destructive to self and to others. In the
past several years, I have accumulated hundreds of descriptions of
Type A individuals as given by their mates. Just the following few illustrate how the inner workings of Type A reactors are viewed by their
significant others.

"My wife is the most confident-acting insecure person I have ever
known."

"He has an office filled with plaques and certificates that document his accomplishments and the applause he has gotten, but he still
feels unappreciated and unrecognized."

"He wakes up scared in the middle of the night, and every morning I have to give him a pep talk. Sometimes I feel like a cheerleader."

"When I hug him, he stiffens. When we make love, either he

doesn't seem to know what to do or he acts like a robot stuck on one speed."

"I can tell when she feels ashamed of herself because she starts to justify and rationalize."

"When he worked for someone else, he lived in fear of his manager's criticism. Now he has his own company, and he lives in fear of his customers' criticism."

"She gets a gleam of joy in her eye whenever she talks about any hard times that friends or even relatives are going through; she's the most competitive person I know."

"Beneath all that control lurks anxiety and a feeling of chaos."

"My husband acts like he couldn't care less about you or what you think, but I'll guarantee you this: If you say anything negative to him about him, he will never forget it and he will never forgive you."

"I just wish she would stop torturing herself by comparing herself to everyone else."

"Relaxing makes her tense. She only acts like she's having fun if she's being stimulated in some new and different way."

"He tries to be a good dad, but his attention span is shorter than my children's."

"My wife lives in a constant state of frustration."

"He's ashamed of how prejudiced he is. Ministers aren't supposed to be that way."

"Being with her is like walking on eggshells. You never know when she's going to break into anger."

"He has learned to come home at a reasonable hour, but he feels guilty unless he's working at something that seems absolutely necessary to get done."

"When I see him with his family, he looks like a desperate little boy hoping to get noticed and patted on the back."

These spouses of Type A's know that Type A's, just like the rest of us, are haunted by inner pains and insecurities and that their behavior often masks their vulnerable feelings. The comments of these spouses serve as a backdrop to the following summaries of the psychological and medical research on the inner workings of Type A personalities. This research collectively suggests that Type A's are both born and made. That is, many of these people seem physically predisposed to respond to the world in this manner, and certain environmental factors can and do complicate this preexisting tendency.

Physical Factors

All Type A's tend to behave in the ways described in the preceding pages, at least to some extent. In a nutshell, this way of reacting could be characterized as reflexive frustration and alarm when faced with stressful stimuli. It is tempting to conclude that these people are just immature and impulsive or that they simply need to learn to be more patient and mellow in their daily life-style, and then all will be well.

However, the issue is not that simple; many Type A individuals are "programmed" in a way that is physically different from Type B individuals. Many Type A's experience physiological responses to stressors that differ from the physical stress reactions of the mellow, Type B personality. It is not just that Type A's are more hardheaded or self-focused; they actually react with a different set of central nervous system responses to the multiple stresses of daily living.

More specifically, contemporary research has clearly documented that, compared with Type B subjects, Type A individuals predictably demonstrate an exaggerated physiological alarm reaction to stressful events, and a very weak physiological calming reaction. Let me explain this extremely important point in understanding why Type A's react as they do.

Stress Reactions

All humans react to stressful events with the activation of the sympathetic or emergency branch of the autonomic nervous system. This sympathetic activity causes a burst of adrenaline and other substances into the body, resulting in the body's kicking into overdrive in preparation for dealing with a stressor. This overdrive prepares the body for fight or flight. It results in various physical and psychological reactions such as increased heart rate, elevated blood pressure, increased muscular tension, and narrowing of psychological focus to the cause of the stress reaction.

To prevent a physiological blowout from continuous activation of this emergency reaction, the autonomic nervous system next switches on the parasympathetic (or calming) branch. This reaction calms and soothes by shutting down the fight-or-flight reaction.

A fascinating and profoundly important point of contemporary research on Type A reactivity is that, *when faced with a stressor, Type A personalities evidence an exaggerated autonomic nervous system alarm reaction and an impoverished calming reaction.*

In stressful situations, in other words, Type A's secrete more adrenaline and experience greater increases in heart rate and blood pressure than Type B's. Type B's, on the other hand, evidence more prolonged and more effective calming-branch autonomic nervous system reactions. No wonder Type A's overreact and find it so difficult to remain cool, calm, and collected during stressful times; they are working with a physiological handicap! This is a vital fact to remember about Type A behavior. This fact is often overlooked in the private struggles of married couples. One of my type A patients lamented:

"My wife, who's the original mellow Earth Mother, just doesn't understand that I can't always help reacting like I do. We can go on a picnic with our kids, and all the way to the park I can remind myself to just cool it, relax, and enjoy being with my family. But when one of the kids spills his drink, or skins his knees playing, or has any of the little emergencies that I know will happen, my first reactions are likely to be overreactions. I just get this burst of tension and urgency inside me that I know my wife doesn't experience. I'm getting better at calming down faster, but I swear I can't seem to control that initial burst!"

The Variety of Type A Reactions

All Type A's do not react to stressors exactly alike. Physical overreactivity does seem to be a general characteristic of Type A's, but some are more reactive than others, and some individuals probably show more reflexive physiological reaction at some times than at other times.

Current research does suggest that certain Type A's do predictably show extreme, reflexive reactivity to any frustrating stimulus. These individuals, who can be referred to as *hot reactor* Type A's, are thought to be the population that is at greatest risk of developing heart disease because of the excessive amounts of physical stress and strain that come from their repeated activation of the flight-or-fight syndrome throughout daily living.

These hot reactors also seem to be the Type A's who experience the greatest marital and family discord, as measured by the evaluations of other family members. Remember, these people are not accurate observers of their own behavior or of the effect their behavior has on others. As a result, they may be only minimally aware of the degree of marital and family distress they are living with. (Just ask their spouses.)

To understand this factor of differing degrees of physiological reactivity found in different personality styles, it is helpful to think in terms of a continuum. At one end of the continuum is the hot reactor Type A. At the other end is the Type B. At various points between lie different combinations of Type A and Type B coping patterns. Experiments have been published that document the varying degrees of physiological reactivity of individuals who fall all along the continuum. For example, if a diversified group of Type A and Type B personalities is monitored for physiological reactions to frustrating stimuli such as noise or an unsolvable math problem, an interesting variation in physical response is seen.

The Type B subjects in such settings show brief elevations in measures of physical alarm and tension. Then they settle down relatively rapidly and adopt the attitude "Now, isn't this interesting? I can't solve this problem." On the other hand, some of the Type A reactors show elevated spikes of physical alarm and tension in response to these stressors, and they remain physically alarmed as they grapple with the problems at hand. Still others, the hot reactor Type A's, spike extremely high and quickly on measures of physical responsivity. Their measures of physical alarm may begin to lower repeatedly, only to spike again. In parallel to these physical responses, the hot reactors grow more angry and frustrated as the urgency of their need to solve the problem mounts. These people often return to the study site a day or so after participating in such experiments, saying, "Give me another chance. I can solve that damned problem today."

Hot Reactors and Relationships

Relationship styles are affected by individual physical reaction patterns. When faced with a frustrating situation, hot reactors seem almost unable to react with calm understanding and tolerance. These are the spouses who yell, get red in the face, exaggerate in the midst of an argument, and negotiate by bullying.

It is important to remember that this initial period of hot reaction is not fully under one's individual control. This statement is not intended to give license to such outbursts, however. If you are a hot reactor, your basic psychological task in life is to learn to control your behavior better in reaction to this physiological burst of alarm. You can do so by following the various suggestions for modifying Type A style that are outlined in chapter 12 and by committing yourself to an overall program of healthy emotional management as discussed in chapter 13.

Following the guidelines in chapters 12 and 13 is essential for a hot reactor Type A; the first step in gaining self-control is to lower baseline levels of stress and tension. Attempting to control yourself in the midst of an alarm reaction is difficult and painful. Do not wait until a storm of hot reactions breaks over you before attempting to change; learn to lower your general tension level so that an occurrence of hot reaction won't push you over the edge of acceptable behavior.

Your alarm reaction will occur reflexively: accept this fact. But the effect of the alarm reaction on your behavior will be lessened if the baseline from which this response originates is lower. Lowering your baseline of tension and stress begins with your willingness to make some commonsense choices in orchestrating the situations that fill your daily life. Here are some examples:

Choose to associate with people who soothe you, not with people who stir your competitive feelings.

Engage in activities that provide you with comfortable degrees of stimulation, not ones that overexcite aggressive and hostile reactions.

Exercise regularly; learn and use a physical relaxation technique to discharge excessive energy and to lower your overall level of physical reactivity.

Practice making a mental note of the effect your behavior has on others.

Practice apologizing when your reactions have hurt or frightened others.

Anticipate your initial period of hot reaction in certain situations coming up (for example, a family trip or a tense business meeting), and count to 450 before responding. (Count slowly, not by 50s!)

If you are the spouse of a hot reactor Type A, you probably spend a great deal of time running interference for your spouse in the hope of fending off an outburst. You also probably are frustrated with your lack of success in running *enough* interference and with your partner's lack of progress in learning to react more calmly. It is important for you to be realistic about your goal here, and about your expectations of your spouse.

Certainly no one has the right to treat another person with hostility and lack of consideration. However, if you are going to remain married to a hot reactor Type A, you must realize that your partner may react with an unfair amount of hostility at times. It may not be fair, but it is a fact.

Try to avoid the traps of developing mutual anger, resentment, and hostile reaction that are outlined in chapter 11, about Type A marital patterns. Many of the spouses of hot reactors whom I have treated refuse to accept the reality that their mates will never turn into Type B personalities, no matter how much preaching, crying, poor health, or negative emotional and relationship consequences come their way.

Be realistic in your expectations. Your partner can and should learn to tone down the hot reactor style, making episodes less intense and, it is hoped, less frequent. But you may also need to change your reactions to your partner's Type A behavior.

Try to avoid conveying condescending judgment of your partner's episodes of hot reaction. Being judged merely fuels the Type A fire. Many Type A's would struggle successfully through episodes of hot reactivity with relatively little interpersonal consequence if their spouses would not convey negative judgment of their actions at the moment. Try not to turn every moment of stressful reaction into an interpersonally stressful event. For example, your hot reactor wife may be cursing at the driver of the car ahead, but there is no need for you to react in a way that generates tension between the two of you.

Let her be angry with the other driver. You have to ride in the car with her, and you deserve to be reasonably comfortable. It is painful enough to witness such an outburst. Do not further your pain, and your partner's, by picking a fight about how she reacted.

In learning to cope better with your own or your partner's Type A style (hot reactor or not), it helps to understand the psychological roots of this personality pattern.

Psychological Roots of Type A-ness

From a psychological perspective, it makes most sense to view the Type A behavior pattern as a general coping response. Research suggests that when Type A's perceive an actual or potential threat to their sense of control, they reflexively begin struggling to regain control. The struggle to regain control leads to the Type A behavior patterns. Type A's in action may look like individuals fighting against invisible challenges and threats to their very survival.

What kinds of life experiences and psychological operations result in such a coping pattern? To answer this question, I first summarize research on the early experiences of Type A individuals. Next I highlight the beliefs that seem to drive Type A behavioral choices. Finally I describe the behavioral and emotional triangle of superperson-depression-anger in which most Type A's live.

Early Life Experiences of Type A's

Is the Type A behavior pattern shaped by certain life experiences that are different from other people's? Many researchers have attempted to answer this question, and the quest for clarity on the issue continues. However, researchers generally agree that Type A behavior probably develops, at least in part, because the childhood environment revolves around the following family patterns:

- Parents are rather unloving and unpredictable in their reactions to the child's behavior.
- Parental approval is given only if the child performs exceptionally.

- Parents pay attention mainly to outcome, or to the product of the child's efforts, rather than respond with affirming attention to the child.

- Parents are extremely critical of any behavior on the part of the child that does not live up to their expectations.

- Parents model behavior for the child and verbally drive the child with messages to be strong, be perfect, try harder, and hurry up.

- One parent may have a stronger influence than the other. Male Type A's may have mothers who delivered the messages and processes described above, and who withheld any unconditional expression of love and affirmation. Female Type A's may have fathers who were critical or absent; the father of a female Type A may also have been a "failed hero" because of his own problems with positive adjustment (for example, he may have been alcoholic or a financial failure, and so on).

In short, researchers suggest that Type A individuals tend to come from families with demanding, critical parents. Type A individuals seem to have had relatively little experience in being unconditionally loved, nurturingly affirmed and soothed, and gently taught necessary lessons, all of which develop a calming sense of mastery in living life.

Remember that these are the same people who are born with an overreactive alarm branch of the central nervous system and an underactive calming nervous system response. This combination of (1) physical predisposition to experience anxiety and agitation and (2) critical family environment is thought to lead to the development of internal negative self-evaluation. Thus is born the Type A individual's greatest secret: at the core of this whirlwind of behavioral action and apparent power lie negative self-esteem and pervasive anxiety.

Of course, the family environment is not totally responsible for personality development. The effects of peers and of such settings as school environments also have much to do with how we learn to cope. It often seems, though, that by secondary school age, the behavior styles that ultimately blossom into Type A syndromes begin to solidify. Type A boys are likely to compensate for an underlying negative sense of self by focusing on achievements—an endeavor that is often blatantly encouraged by society in general, regardless of what is happening at home. Early in life, such kids begin what will develop into a chronic struggle to do more than time allows. This hurry sickness may increase the sense of urgency that underlies the eventual development of the aggressive, free-floating hostility that many Type A's eventually demonstrate.

The process of development that begins with secondary school is thought to be somewhat different for Type A girls. The developing female Type A is thought to channel her internal struggle for approval into succeeding in friendship circles. Most females are discouraged by society from showing aggressive, openly competitive behavior. Many such children therefore learn to channel this energy into what may become a competitive quest to be perfectly popular with peers and to become the perfect caretaker of others' needs. Unfortunately, the standards of evaluating success in being a caretaker are not clear; no trophies or report cards are given for this activity. Lack of clear validation of the female Type A's efforts adds more fuel to stress. Time urgency and increased irritability come when the Type A girl adds school, work, and other nonrelationship responsibilities to her overall load of performance pressures. As will be discussed in chapter 10, Type A-ness presents special problems for contemporary women, the majority of whom feel driven by an overwhelming combination of relationship and work stressors.

Much of this characterization of how the Type A behavior pattern develops is speculative. Many Type A's come from families that are quite different from any that have been described. Furthermore, many individuals go through family and life experiences of the sorts that have been mentioned *without* developing this pattern of coping.

Two general points emerge from this discussion. First, I strongly believe that insecurity and anxiety—not anger, grandiosity, or confidence—are the factors that underlie the Type A style of coping. Second, the interplay between physiological reactivity and psychosocial experiences is central in the development of Type A behavior pattern.

Beliefs That Drive Type A Behavior

It is little wonder that Type A's, having had such life experiences, develop a rather hostile, guarded, and emotionally cautious way of viewing the world. These negative attitudes complicate the already existing physical difficulties that these people have in relaxing. They often learn to fear that bad things will happen if they do relax.

In general, Type A's are driven by the belief that they must constantly prove themselves. This quest is usually fueled by an unconscious sense of negative self-esteem, which probably has much to do with the competitive defensiveness that typifies so many of the Type A interpersonal reactions.

Both negative self-esteem and Type A behavior are fueled by the beliefs that form these peoples' attitudes. Type A beliefs and their subsequent behavior patterns are summarized in table 10.2. As you can see from the table, beliefs born from insecurities fuel Type A reactivity. The behavior of a Type A person is powerful, but underlying this display of power are haunting insecurities and ways of thinking. This way of being leads to painful struggles that take various forms, as will be seen in the following pages.

The Type A Triad

Researcher Virginia Price has proposed that Type A's tend to shift around among three distinct psychological postures, which consist of certain cognitive, behavioral, and physiological characteristics. The three most frequent Type A states are the *Superperson* state, the *Depressed* state, and the *Angry* state.[12]

The Superperson State

This is the driven way of living in which most Type A's spend most of their time, struggling to prove to an imaginary audience that they are

[12]V. Price, *Type A Behavior Pattern*, p. 180–90, with permission.

Table 10.2 Type A Beliefs and Behaviors

Believing that . . .	The type A acts . . .
"I must constantly prove myself,"	as if life is an endless struggle.
"My sense of well-being is always in jeopardy,"	on guard and defensive.
"Others can take away my self-worth,"	hostile.
"I am not as good as others,"	competitive and jealous and critical of self and of others.
"I am not as talented as others,"	as if he or she must always try harder than others.
"Good may not prevail in the world,"	suspicious of the intentions of others.
"All resources are scarce,"	urgently competitive.

worthy of high regard. Here, it is as though the Type A is saying to the world, "I'm proving myself as fast as I can." While operating in this state, Type A's often juggle several major tasks or projects. The accomplishment of one goal simply leads them to switch focus to the next goal or project.

As described by Price, the Superperson state is characterized by extreme amounts of the following attributes: "high performance standards, superabundant energy, extreme ambitiousness, exceptionally hard-driving effort, super-efficiency, super-conscientiousness, extreme competence and ingenuity, excessive competitiveness, hyper-alertness, excessive haste, chronic high levels of activity, and super-aggressiveness" (p. 182).

In this state, Type A's become excessively focused on pursuing goals. Time is structured and energies are expended with a relentless degree of drive. At such times, Type A's may simply not notice environmental stimuli that are unrelated to the task at hand. Type A Superpersons fail to monitor signs of increasing mental or physical fatigue and may fail to notice the negative impact that this mode of living is having on their interpersonal relationships. This way of living understandably leads to increased fatigue and tension for Type A's. They eventually begin to show signs of emotional and physical burnout. As this burnout begins, they become particularly sensitive to any negative events in their lives.

Accordingly, Superperson Type A's usually fall into the second stage of the Type A triad—the Depressed state—in reaction to such events as failing to meet perfectionistic standards; being criticized by others (by an enraged spouse who is tired of being neglected, for example); getting physically sick from the wear and tear of living under such prolonged stress; or any unexpected life trauma (for example, a spouse's illness).

The Depressed State

Type A's run hard and crash harder. Many researchers consider depression to be the flip side of the Type A behavior complex. This is understandable when you consider how unnurturing and joyless life becomes from prolonged states of Superperson Type A living.

While operating in the Depressed state, Type A's become overwhelmed with self-blame and discouragement. They are paralyzed by the fear that they may never be able to overcome the many obstacles that they perceive to be in their path. Life can become filled with some or all of the following symptoms for Depressed Type A's: feelings of gloom, of being burdened by life and of being overwhelmed; guilt about the impact that their behavior during the Superperson flurry has had on others; low energy, lack of pleasurable reactions, sleep disturbance, or various physical problems that become the focus of obsession and shame and embarrassment over experiencing any of the above.

Type A's have particular difficulty coping with depression for three reasons. First, when depressed, they are unable to engage in their typical mode of defending themselves from awareness of their underlying low self-esteem—their Superperson behavior. Their depression is thus fueled by the surfacing of overwhelmingly negative self-evaluations when they slow down, exhausted from the prior Superperson flurry. Second, Type A's interpret the surfacing of vulnerable feelings as indicative of weakness. They then become even more self-critical. Third, being rather distrustful of the good intentions of others in the first place (remember table 10.2?) they then tend to project their negative self-judgments onto others; they fear that they will be criticized by others if they let their pain be known. They may begin to avoid others, thereby increasing their own sense of isolation. In this manner, depression escalates. The depression continues until Type A's do one of two things: (1) once physical energy is regained from the "rest" that came with slowing down while depressed, Type A's may distract themselves from further depression by switching back into the Superperson state, this time geared with even higher goals and even greater urgency (both of which are now needed in order to overcome the elevated level of depression); or (2) they may move into the Angry state.

The Angry State

Being angry hurts less than being sad. Type A's know this better than most people. Becoming Angry is the inevitable consequence of the Type A's tendency to project self-blaming intentions onto others when feeling vulnerable. In doing so, Type A's externalize their own anger or disappointment with themselves by assigning responsibility for their pain to someone or something else. In this manner, anger toward others helps reduce anger toward self.

My impression is that Type A personalities accumulate such a wealth of experience with this form of transfer of feelings that they eventually become stuck in the following pattern of feelings substitution: any surfacing of self-doubt or feelings of vulnerability, which might otherwise trigger depressive reactions, triggers Angry reactions instead. The next step is to find a person, event, or obstacle on which to vent this anger.

Price says that this Angry state of Type A functioning "is characterized by self-justification and by accusation of others. Self-righteous demeanor (i.e., I am right and you are wrong), interpersonal tension, impatience, intolerance, and sudden bursts of anger, or even rage, can also be observed. . . . Persons in the angry state often report feeling victimized and, therefore, justified in insuring that justice occurs; that is, they seek revenge" (p. 189).

Unfortunately, family members are often the targets of the angry projections that characterize the Type A's switching from the Depressed state to the Angry state. I often see Type A heart patients who are momentarily soothing their depression by blaming their spouses, children, relatives, employers, or anyone who will slow down long enough to be identified.

Because this wild person state of Type A reaction is so frightening, loved ones of such a person sometimes have difficulty remembering that this behavior is being fueled by fear and by a flight from depression. Running from discomfort eventually leads Type A's to gear up again for another major Superperson burst of activity—taking up a new hobby, buying a new house, starting a new business—anything to avoid depression. Cycling back and forth from Superperson state to Angry state is the way many Type A's live. Such a life-style has understandable negative effects on marriage and family life.

Summary

Unchecked Type A behavior is not only uncomfortable, it is dangerous. Both for individuals and for couples, the consequence of letting this way of reacting run wild is damage to health.

Changing this coping pattern begins with accepting that Type A reactions (1) have to do with both physical and psychological responses, (2) are efforts to regain or maintain control, and (3) mask underlying feelings of insecurity. Because Type A reactions disrupt marital intimacy in predictable ways unless controlled, it is important to accept these facts and begin developing alternate ways of responding to stress. Guidelines for individuals and couples who want to make such changes are offered in the following chapters.

Eleven

Living with Type A's

This is a test; complete this sentence. I am married to a Type A personality, and I: (1) am Type A myself; (2) frequently compete with my mate, even when I don't want to; (3) wish that my partner would be more relaxed and nurturing in dealing with me and the kids; (4) am convinced that my mate is acting more and more like my mother-in-law (father-in-law); (5) feel very, very tired; (6) wish I could get my mate to read this book; (7) am filled with fear and anticipation as I read on.

As your answers to this test may indicate, Type A people can be difficult to live with. Of the many Type A factors described in the preceding pages, few have desirable effects on relationships. This is somewhat unfair to us Type A's; we do have our charming moments. In fact, healthily refined Type A's are typically quite enjoyable and stimulating to be around—when their lives are going well.

The situation relevant to this book, however, is one in which the Type A's life is not going so well. Coping with heart disease is frightening, and (as we all know by now) when Type A's get scared, they go into action or become angry. For this reason, when at least one member of a cardiac couple is Type A, the couple's relationship can be quite affected by the negative aspects of this coping style.

Marriages tend to organize around the couple's most consistent behavioral and emotional ways of being, so it is no wonder that Type A coping style tends to shape marital interactions. This Type A business is not subtle; its power and effect on others are quite obvious.

Of course, a number of factors in addition to Type A behavior combine to determine how a couple acts. These factors include the emotional histories of the individuals and of the relationship; the overall stress level of the family; whether both spouses are Type A; and the relative levels of love, commitment, and forgiveness in the relationship. As was pointed out in chapter 7, these factors certainly influ·nce the overall quality of the marriage, and their importance should not be discounted.

An extensive discussion of all the factors affecting marital development is beyond the scope of this book. But understanding the range of pitfalls that can occur in Type A marriages *is* within the scope of this book, and understanding these pitfalls can help you understand your reactions to heart illness.

Research suggests that marriages that are dominated by one partner's Type A style tend to have serious problems, particularly from the viewpoint of the non–Type A spouse. For example, wives of male Type A's frequently report feelings of depression, worthlessness, anxiety, and tension. They also tend to feel more guilt and social isolation than spouses of Type B personalities. Various complaints of women married to Type A men have repeatedly surfaced in research studies, including resentment over their absence from home, frustration with their failure to help with at-home chores, and criticism of their lack of parenting abilities and generally poor communication and conflict resolution skills. Very little research attention has been paid, on the other hand, to the reaction of men to their Type A wives. Preliminary studies suggest that Type A male cardiac patients have a better recovery rate if they are married to nurturing, Type B women than if they are married to Type A wives. I emphasize that these findings are speculative and tentative. Don't run out and get divorced in the name of cardiac rehabilitation! Read on and learn how to make your relationship an asset in your rehabilitation.

A fair amount of recent research attention has been paid to the Type A pattern as it occurs in women. More and more women in our culture are displaying Type A characteristics, a phenomenon that is certainly related to the increased complexity of contemporary female roles. More than 50 percent of American women now work outside the home, and approximately 44 percent of all women in the United States with school-age children are employed. Studies have shown that, for most women, employment outside the home does not lessen perceived or actual responsibility for running the household and performing domestic tasks; women just add employment to their other responsibilities. One study reported that employed women spend as many as 80 to 120 hours a week working in their combined domestic and career roles.

The result is increased time urgency, irritability, reactivity to stress, and feelings of urgency about the need to control one's environment. Such women also tend to drive themselves with perfectionistic demands to ensure that their spouses and children suffer no inconveniences because of their career involvements. In short, such women are at risk of escalating Type A patterns as their lives become more complex.

Most spouses of Type A persons (even spouses who are Type A themselves) worry about the effect their mates' Type A reactivity will have on their children. And well they should. Type A individuals do tend to parent in ways that foster Type A reactions in children:

They react to children's behavior more often with critical comments than with nurturing and praising comments.

Then tend to perceive children as stressors.

They often feel that they lack (and sometimes they do lack) skills needed to communicate effectively with and deal with children.

They tend to project their own insecurities onto their children, conveying the message that the children need to perform well enough to make up for their lack of self-esteem.

Such parenting can damage children's self-esteem. But even if a couple's children have healthy and positive personalities, many aspects of the Type A behavior pattern can result in lessened marital and family intimacy. For example, the overstressed Type A spouse may not notice or remember the details of the family's daily or weekly activities, like a wife's medical appointment or a son's math test. As a result, the Type A might simply forget to inquire about or comment on how things are going in the other person's life.

The Type A's own high standards of performance and shaky self-esteem might lead to undue embarrassment over the physical appearance or behaviors of loved ones—as if their characteristics or actions were somehow a reflection of the Type A's personal worth. The result is a critical approach rather than a nurturing, supportive approach to the family.

The Type A's hard-driving style may interfere with smelling-the-roses experiences that create intimacy and connection among family members. Or competitiveness may lead the Type A to hold back statements of praise and appreciation for the accomplishments of other family members. Aggressive, hostile reactions from the Type A make it difficult to resolve conflict successfully, and family members may begin to distance themselves from this person because they fear having another no-winners argument.

The Type A's time urgency may turn even supposedly relaxed events, like evenings when the couple goes out for a date, into tense, scheduled occasions that are more endured than enjoyed. And the Type A's extreme discomfort with lack of control often makes the whole realm of interpersonal relations—with all its infinite and wonderful sloppiness—an arena to be avoided or, at best, struggled with.

Despite these universals, no single pattern of relating exists in Type A marriages. I doubt that any such universal pattern will ever be discovered, because every person (even one who has most of the defining characteristics of a certain personality label) is unique. However, in my work as a marriage therapist, I have noted seven styles of relating within marriages in which partners are grappling with Type A behavior. One of these may be considered a healthy version of marriage; the other patterns surely result in increased stress and dissatisfaction within the marriage. I offer these descriptions to you in hopes of stimulating your thinking and your discussions about yourselves and your own marital patterns.

I emphasize that the following conceptualizations are the result of one person's clinical impressions of and review of contemporary research on Type A behavior and marriage. Although research in this area has been rather limited, my clinical experiences have been extensive and varied. I also emphasize that my conceptualizations of marital types do not represent absolute, mutually, exclusive marital patterns.

Many couples display several of these patterns of interaction, and no couple totally fits any one of these descriptions.

The "Good Mother–Bad Boy" Type A Pattern

This is perhaps the classic Type A marriage, the form that predominated before so many women joined the Type A ranks in contemporary times. A Type A man selects a Good Mother (usually a Type B) whose gentle and patient manner carries with it the promise of the unconditional nurturance that was lacking in his upbringing. Such a woman has usually been brought up to be a gentle caretaker. She is driven by a Pleasing Others old-brain message (see chapter 9). Her Type A spouse's need for nurturance therefore fits nicely with her own personality dynamics.

Such couples typically develop a fairly traditional division of roles. The man earns the money, or the bulk of it, by working at a stressful job that requires considerable absence from home. In his absence, the wife takes over the multiple tasks involved in running the household and family. She parents the children, cooks and cleans, and generally runs the couple's domestic life.

The wife also functions as the stress absorber in the system; she is the family member in charge of soothing everyone else when nerves get jangled. She is also in charge of praising others to bolster their self-esteem. These women are often treated like junior business partners by their dominating Type A husbands. They are respected, but they are not recognized as equal in power to the big boss.

Such couples live with the underlying hope—and sometimes the openly expressed plan—that the woman's nurturing ways will gradually change the man's Type A tendencies. It is as though these couples had adopted a contract stating that the Type A spouse has simply not yet been loved and nurtured enough in his life to blossom into a mellow Type B personality, and that the woman's job in this marriage is to love her Bad Boy in ways that will change him into a patient, tolerant, relaxed, noncompetitive individual.

Guess what happens next.

Actually, this contract is sometimes fulfilled to a degree. Some

Type A's do learn from the example (or perhaps from the exasperation) of their Type B mates. However, far more often both spouses in this relationship category end up feeling rather disillusioned and double-crossed because the original plan does not come true.

The woman in such a relationship often begins to grow tired of her subordinate position in the marriage and frustrated that her good loving is not changing the Bad Boy at all. He continues in his Type A ways and may even become increasingly Type A as the stress of mid-life approaches. She may gradually grow resentful about her relative lack of validation and recognition. The importance of her role in life and in the family may go unnoticed versus the glory claimed by and given to her husband for being the financial head of the household. She also may begin to feel neglected by her mate, who seldom notices or understands all she does to manage her share of their collective load. It is clear in such marriages that the man's stress is considered the more painful, and he is therefore treated as the partner more deserving of special attention and rest.

As time passes, the Type A husband in such a marriage typically reports a longing for the good old days when he had his wife's undivided attention and unending tolerance. He may have difficulty sharing this nurturing mother with others, even with their own children. He may also have much difficulty understanding his spouse's pain and her disillusionments with their marriage. Remember, Type A's have trouble seeing their impact on others. Such a man tends to attribute his wife's growing negative feelings to her excessive worrying about the kids, about her own parents, or about his health. It seldom dawns on him that the woman might be feeling depressed because of what she is not getting from him.

An interesting next step often seen in the operations of such couples is that the Type A man begins expressing anger with his wife because she is no longer as nurturing as she used to be. He is especially likely to accuse her of being unnurturing during a period when he has taken particularly poor care of himself with reference to stress management. In other words, he may work himself into feeling exhausted, isolated, and somewhat depressed and then blame these feelings on his wife. The amazing thing is that the wife often believes this criticism.

The wife often accepts the blame because of her own feelings of guilt, which have developed because she is aware of feeling resentful. Remember, feeling angry is not acceptable to a person who is driven by a Pleasing Others personality. Plus, the emotional "contract" did specify that she would be the never-ending source of nurturing in this marriage. If he is unhappy, it must be because she is not taking appropriate care of him; therefore, she must deserve the blame that he is dishing out.

These marriages typically function relatively smoothly for quite a while. The division of labors and responsibilities works well enough to maintain a functional balance in day-to-day living. However, this same division of life involvements tends to lead eventually to the sense of living separate lives. The couple may have totally separate friendship groups, interests, passions, and so on. They may share very few interests except on an abstract level. For example, he might vehemently express a shared concern for and interest in their kids but actually have little working knowledge of or involvement in their daily lives. She might express respect for and interest in his work but actually be rather bored with it.

At this point many such women go to their physicians complaining of vague physical ailments, or to counselors for help in feeling happier. These women have difficulty accepting that their feelings of discontent in their marriages are well justified. They therefore often mask these negative feelings by focusing on other physical or emotional concerns. In living as caretakers of others' needs, they have grown accustomed to discounting their own emotional needs. They often lament, "I should be happier. I have everything I ever wanted. What's wrong with me? Maybe I just need to grow up."

Maybe so. But such a woman also probably needs to come to grips, along with her mate, with the frustrating aspects of their marriage. The problem is that such honest coming to grips probably means giving the Type A spouse feedback that he does not want to hear, and examining her own frustrations and fears in a way that flies in the face of her Pleasing Others coping style.

One frequent realization of such a woman is the fear that her own caretaking behavior may, in fact, be enabling rather than modifying her husband's Type A patterns: As long as she plays the role of stress absorber, he may have less need to learn to manage stress for himself. As long as she serves as the sole nurturer in the family, he need not learn how to be more nurturing of others. As long as she keeps forgiving him for his many Type A transgressions, he may never change. The worried wife may check out this fear of enabling with her Type A husband, only to be assured by him that he would only be lost, and worse in his Type A-ness, if she did not nurture him so. (He's no fool; why change a good thing?)

For such a marriage to grow, at first the wife has to push for changes that the Type A husband will probably resist. Even though doing so goes much against the grain of her Pleasing Others personality, she must keep pushing for a healthier way of relating, rather than settle into forever being a partner in her mate's Type A dance.

Finally, I want to mention a factor that is very much hidden beneath the surface in many of these marriages. As much as they truly value their Good Mother wives, many male Type a's are haunted by a growing degree of boredom with their mates because they have locked in a limited perspective of them, seeing only their nurturing, tolerant, gentle side. Of course, according to the original contract, these wives often show only their Good Mother aspects in the marriage; they express the more spontaneous, earthy, and fun-loving parts of themselves only in friendships or other siblinglike relationships.

The risk of extramarital involvements is relatively high for such couples. Because they grow apart in their lives, both of them become vulnerable to the infatuating experience of finding a soul mate—a member of the opposite sex whose values, interests, and styles of responding to the world more closely match and more directly validate their own way of being.

The "Pleasing Others Even If It Kills Me" Pattern

Here, the marriage is dominated by a person who is not only scripted to Please Others but is Type A to boot. Unlike the women in the Good Mother–Bad Boy Type A pattern, who are Type B caretakers, the caretaker in this marriage is a driven Type A individual. I have observed this pattern in both sexes, but women are more often the enactors of this role.

These women are stuck in a role that can be both exhausting and depressing. They try to be all things to all people and are haunted by perfectionistic standards in all that they attempt. For such women, it isn't enough to have an active career, do all their own domestic work ("I don't need any help; I'm a *real woman*"), and attend all their children's extracurricular activities. They also have to keep up with other parents who are volunteering to help in the school cafeteria and lead the Girl Scout troop. The result? An overwhelming load of responsibilities.

These women are driven by the notion that what others think of them is all that matters. The problem is that this notion applies to everyone in their lives: spouse, children, parents, employers, employees, friends, and acquaintances. Having an inner sense of self that is less than clear, the Pleasing Others Type A wife uses this psychological game plan: "If I do what pleases others, then they will approve of me and I will feel whole inside." These women depend on approval from others to soothe their internal sense of inferiority.

Problems arise in the life of Pleasing Others Type A's if they marry other Type A's (which they often do), and particularly if they marry Type A's who are not Pleasing Others oriented (which they usually are not). The reasons for this matching are logical. Type A's may be attracted to each other by the excitement they feel from the cumulative high energy and intense stimulation of being together. The classic Type A's are also most comfortable with others who defer to their own judgments, thereby giving them a sense of superiority and power. In these marriages the Pleasing Others Type A wife often allows her career and nonfamily involvements to take a back seat to her husband's. In such marriages wife seems to have two choices: depression or stress.

Many women of this personality type choose to give up thriving careers to satisfy their mates' need for full-time nurturers. Of course, such women may also discontinue career pursuits out of a healthy decision to focus on child rearing and domestic aspects of their lives, and not only to give in to a husband's expectations. In either case, though, trouble starts if applause for the Type A wife's efforts stops. Remember,

Type A people need recognition. Housework, carpooling, cooking, and cleaning may not result in enough positive reinforcement to soothe the Type A wife's jangled nerves.

Add to this picture a Type A husband who is rather egocentric, and the progression toward depression escalates for the Pleasing Others Type A woman, such as Gretchen, who has lost the stimulation of a career. Consulting me for treatment of depression, Gretchen openly expressed this dilemma:

"My husband has become powerful and successful in the past thirteen years, and I know I have much to do with that. We've been married for sixteen years, and I've run his life—other than his insurance agency.

"What gets me is this: he has gradually begun treating me like I have no brains. Just because my days are filled with diapers and station wagons loaded with kids, he seems to have forgotten that there are other aspects of me. When we first met, he was trying to figure out what he was going to be when and if he grew up. On the other hand, I had already been named teacher of the year twice in four years. I was a hot shot! He seems to have forgotten that. I seem to forget it myself, more often than not. No wonder I'm depressed; my husband has forgotten who I am and so have I."

Of course, not all Pleasing Others Type A women choose to give up their careers. As mentioned earlier, almost half the mothers in the United States work outside the home now. But working outside the home just adds to the stress in the lives of these women and further complicates their coping struggles.

Couples caught in this brand of Type A marriage inevitably suffer from the exhaustion that comes from what is often a joint quest to do it all at a level of 110 percent. As fatigue sets in, the couple begin neglecting to attend to each other in an intimate and nurturing manner. Such couples develop marriages that are characterized by fatigue rather than lively intimacy.

The "Ready, Set, Go!" Pattern

This is the pattern that emerges when two exceptionally competitive Type A's marry. This pattern is often manifested by dual-career couples, though I have also noticed it in couples who live on only one income.

The meaning of life in this type of marriage seems to be competition. These partners compete both openly and subtly. They may make mental or verbal comparisons regarding anything and everything: how much money each one earns, who's in better physical condition, who's a better tennis player, who's more or less Type A, or who has the better relationship with the children. Because they both are so addicted to stimulation, they tend to fill their lives with activity. They even choose vacations that involve high levels of stimulation rather than relaxation.

I have noticed an interesting result of this kind of competition. When the Type A man is in some way losing in the overall competition for status and power in the marriage, he sometimes one-ups his mate by becoming intent on developing a more nurturing relationship with the children than the wife has. Because the Type A woman is driven to do all things perfectly, including being the perfect mother, such a development in her family fuels her insecurity and drivenness.

With all this competition and frenzied pace of living, no one is available in these marriages to act as stress absorber and nurturer to the other mate. These couples therefore sometimes settle into a suffering contest. Interactions revolve around indirect requests for support and nurturance. Conversation becomes filled with complaints about busy schedules, fatigue, and stress. Power struggles often result over who will grace the other with relief of domestic responsibilities so there will be some free time for doing more work or for trying to recover from another exhausting week. Because both spouses end up feeling similar degrees of stress, a spouse who grants such nurturing breaks does so at the expense of perpetuating his or her own exhaustion. Often, neither spouse has the energy to give the other a nurturing break.

These couples live out the Type A stress nightmare that, indeed, there is not enough nurturing, love, time, attention, or resources in general to go around. During their frequent periods of exhaustion, such couples tend to long for a simpler life. They harbor fantasies of slowing down and quitting their high-stress jobs, buying a small country store (or an equivalent fantasy), and settling for less "stuff" so they will have more time to live. However, each assumes that the other would never be satisfied with such a life. Actually, probably neither one would be. As one such woman once told me, "Sure, we might buy that little country store and enjoy that life for a while. But after six months, one or the other of us would be talking about opening a franchise of these little, relaxing places. I guarantee it."

This longing for more soothing nurturing in life sometimes gets displaced onto others, leading to the development of infatuations with strong, nurturing-seeming members of the opposite sex. Such seemingly Good Mother (or Good Father) types represent a solution to the Type A's drivenness: the possibility of securing help in developing a more comfortable balance in life. The risk of infatuation is particularly high if the other person's style conveys both nurturance and a little bit of feistiness; too much gentleness may be too boring a contrast to the frantic pace that has become a habit for Type A's who have lived in this form of marriage.

The "Chaotic Desperation" Pattern

Stressful as life is for the competitive couples just described, for turmoil and eventual despair they do not even compare with the people caught in this next pattern of Type A marriage. These are the ones whose marriages revolve around a hot reactor Type A personality (see chapter 10) and are affected by the frequent bursts of extreme behavior that characterize Type A hot reactivity. These bursts can involve anger, activity, blame, or substance abuse, to name but a few possibilities.

The destructive impact of such outbursts and behavioral extremes on a marriage is obvious; they batter its emotional core. These extreme events often lead to an emotional shutdown in the marriage or to defensive and bitter conflict that creates distance between spouses. Remaining emotionally open simply begins to feel too risky when your mate might explode into painful anger or activity at any moment.

When the spouse withdraws emotionally, the desperation and fears that underlie the hot reactor's style become fuel injected. Herein lies the great paradox of this version of Type A reactivity: these seemingly self-focused and individualistic hot reactors, who apparently work hard to avoid intimacy in their lives, are often desperately dependent on getting nurturing input from their spouses. Such Type A's often fear their own self-destructiveness deeply. They are anxious about whether they will be capable of holding themselves together for another day of struggles and battles with the outside world. They feel as though life is filled with demons, both internal and external, and that moments of loving connection with their spouses are the only soothing experiences available in their lives.

If the mate of a hot reactor Type A is a Type B personality, this mate often drifts into a state of depression over being unable to change the hot reactor's coping style. Enduring becomes the meaning of life, and emotional shutdown helps us endure. When the mate begins to act depressed, the Type A spouse often feels guilty: "Look what I've done now with my disgusting self. I'm ruining my spouse's life." Or the Type A spouse might escape despair by fleeing into anger: "I've got enough problems without you guilt-tripping me and accusing me of being the source of your pain."

If the mate is also a hot reactor Type A, look out! These are the marriages that frequently explode, either verbally or physically. Many such couples engage in open war by purposely withholding affection and attention, all the while knowing that doing so drives the mate crazy. Peter, a hot reactor patient of mine, explained:

"I work eighteen hours a day, six days a week, and I feel there's nothing I can't accomplish as long as one thing happens: I need my wife to be nice to me in the mornings before I go out to battle the lions. [Note the Superperson state and the paradox of independence and dependence.]

"The problem is that she loves to kick me when I'm down. I was in the middle of closing the biggest deal of my career last month, and sometimes I had to sleep at the office. I would call her in the mornings or drop by to say hello before the new day's battle began, and she wouldn't even kiss me or tell me she loved me! When she acts like that, I go into a rage that ruins my entire morning. I don't understand why she won't understand how important it is for her to be nice to me! After all, I'm doing all this work to provide a good life for her and for our kids." [Note the denial of responsibility for self, projection of blame, and unawareness of the impact of his own behaviors on the emotions of others.]

These couples truly do live in a state of chaos and desperation. They feel trapped by their fears of destruction. The hot reactor fears being destroyed if he or she is not loved back, and the mate shares this fear. These are the people who often lament, "I can't live with you, and I can't live without you."

The "Island Man/Woman" Pattern

In contrast to the chaotic emotional connections in hot reactor marriages, the next pattern is characterized by extremes of emotional and behavioral detachment and disconnection. Here, life revolves around the Type A who conveys the attitude "What I think, need, or want is all that really matters. Other people are an inconvenience to be endured." Such people become extremely self-focused and isolated, appearing to pay no attention to feedback from others about their behavior. They seem no more than slightly irritated when spouse or family complain that they want more emotional connection from them.

These people are excessively demanding of themselves, and they tend to live lives filled with self-disciplined pursuit of their lofty goals. In so doing, they ask for and expect very little support from others. They appear independent, aloof, or even arrogant in their approach to life.

This lack of involvement with others is fueled by the belief, conveyed both directly and indirectly, that other people are basically incompetent. For example, when the mate shares details of the upcoming day, this person may respond by quizzing the mate about taking necessary precautions ("Did you remember to fill the car with gas?")

or giving parentlike reminders ("Of course, you'll remember to pick up the dry cleaning on the way home?"). These people simply do not trust others to behave perfectly enough. For example, a banker friend of mine has an Island Woman Type A wife who routinely reviews his balancing of the checkbook; she does not trust her banker husband to add and substract correctly.

This combination of aloofness and faultfinding is a wall that prevents the development or maintenance of intimacy in the marriage. Spouses of such Type A's often come for counseling, requesting help in their painful grapplings with the decision whether to remain in the marriage. These spouses have often been forced to the conclusion that their mates will never change because they are unwilling to do so. Their own depression is related to the lack of intimacy in their lives, and they feel compelled to do something to fix the situation. They know that without the cooperation of their mates, increasing intimacy in the marriage is impossible. They also have learned to fear that their mates will not cooperate in creating more intimacy. This explains why they begin to consider leaving the relationship.

Often, a painful bond in such marriages comes from the spouse's true concern for the seemingly invincible mate. These spouses have occasionally witnessed the Island crumble into depression, having failed to attain the perfectionistic standards that fuel this coping style. Island spouses are also painfully aware of their mates' extreme isolation. They often fear that if they do leave the marriage, the mates will have no anchor during the periodic storms of depression that inevitably batter all islands.

Paralysis, "stuck-ness," quiet desperation, loneliness—all these descriptions apply to this marital pattern.

The "Too Mellow to Admit It" Pattern

Question: As we enter the 1990s, who is closer to fifty years old than to twenty?

Answer: People who were in their twenties during the 1960s.

Question: Who was taught that characteristics such as aggressiveness, competitiveness, hostility, and being in a hurry are particularly undesirable?

Answer: Same as for the first question.

We have a whole new generation of Type A's now, all of whom have an added problem in coping with this syndrome: they have been taught to feel ashamed of themselves. This new generation has heard and read about the risks involved in being Type A, and the warnings have fueled the messages that lingered in their minds from the 1960s about valuing the nonmaterialistic aspects of life, taking time to enjoy life, and so on. They were taught to strive to be Type B.

One couple I treat in marital therapy—both of whom are in their early forties and both of whom are decidedly Type A in their coping style—have the following quote from Oliver Wendell Holmes taped to their refrigerator door: "Nothing is so vulgar as to be in a hurry." As the husband in this couple laughingly explained, "We glance at that old saying every morning as we're rushing around like maniacs, trying to get our kids out the door so we can both zoom to our offices, work like mules all day, rush home, and be reminded every time we go to the fridge that we're really cool because we don't believe in rushing. What a joke."

Such folks often remind me of Type A's with the brakes on. These people, unlike some of the other Type A patterns, do aspire to be more Type B in reaction style, and they judge Type A characteristics negatively. Accordingly, they often fill their free time with supposedly Type B stuff, like attending dance theater productions or symphony concerts. Their secret is that they usually are bored at such events and feel like leaving at intermission.

They also try to squelch their competitiveness, not wanting to appear to stoop to the low levels of comparing their own income or possessions with those of an old classmate. These people usually have also learned to interact with others in a socially skilled manner, perhaps through on-the-job training in effective communication skills. Their secret Type A-ness therefore often goes undetected by others. But of course the secret *is* detected by—who do you suppose? Hint: the answer begins with an *s* and rhymes with *house*. (If you guessed *spouse*, you are either Type A, the spouse of a Type A, or an attentive reader.)

The problem in these marriages is the disdain that one or both spouses have for being Type A. In some of the other patterns of marital relating, this factor of negative judgment about the rightness or wrongness of being a Type A reactor is absent. In those patterns, even though the individuals involved may lament the inconveniences or negative emotional consequences of being married to a Type A mate, the mate's way of coping is not condemned. No judgment is made that being this way is crass, undesirable, unattractive, and appropriate only for people who know less and are less psychologically healthy than others. Rather than shame the Type A spouse, these couples openly label, discuss, and struggle with the Type A coping pattern.

The important word in the preceding sentence is *openly*. In the Mellow Type A marriage, on the other hand, the Type A struggles are more covert; the couple tries to keep the Type A-ness a secret. Keeping an ongoing Type A struggle secret from the outside world is difficult enough, but such couples also tend to try to mask Type A reactions in their private dealings with each other. They do so to avoid being the target of each other's disgust and criticism.

Learning to curb Type A reactivity by practicing new behaviors within the safe privacy of one's marriage is certainly not a bad thing to do. In fact, as I discuss in the following pages, this is the very strategy I recommend for trying to modify Type A coping pattern. In the Mellow Type A marriage, however, the attempts to change Type A reactions are not made in a nurturing spirit of working together to enhance wellness; they come from a shame-based message that says, "Being this way is disgusting, and I am embarrassed by your [or my own] Type A behavior."

The result of the Mellow pattern is increased discontent and struggle in the marriage. As we grow older, it is only natural for us to tire of efforts to change what seem to be our most natural and authentic ways of being. This is true for all personality types, not just Type A's. During adult stages of psychological development, we progress toward more open and authentic expression of our innermost sense of self.

This normal psychological developmental process collides with the "You should be ashamed of yourself" message that is at the root of the Mellow Type A marital pattern. Mellow Type A marriages tend to perpetuate the brand of mid-life crisis that has to do with developing urgent intolerance for "faking it anymore in my life." Type A's living in such marriages may begin to feel trapped and constrained by the marriages, which do not fit their most natural way of being.

Again, I want to clarify that this pattern does *not* involve the Type A's romanticizing or endorsing all the manifestations of Type A behavior. To the contrary, this new generation of Type A's probably values Type B reactivity more than does any other version of Type A personality.

What grows intolerable to such individuals is the rigid criticism coming from the other spouse. Such criticism is often fueled by the spouse's own, even more secretive and shameful grapplings with Type A syndrome. The message given by such a person often sounds to a marital therapist like, "I want my mate to change all that disgusting Type A stuff so that my own Type A reactions will calm down and I'll never have to confront myself about this same issue."

With this secretive struggle and all these negative judgments floating around in the marriage, many of these seemingly Mellow couples develop a very bitter and blatantly Type A flavor. These couples often settle into a style of living that is all about trying really hard not to try so hard.

The "Using Our Good Stuff to Make It Better" Pattern

All is not bleak for Type A couples. There certainly is such a person as a healthy Type A individual, and many healthy Type A marriages exist. These are the people who collectively use their considerable resources to create thriving, productive lives and intimate, stimulating marriages.

In presenting workshops about how to modify dysfunctional Type A characteristics, I always challenge the participants to begin using their wealth of psychological and physical horsepower to create a higher quality of life. A Type A person who accepts this challenge inevitably begins truly to change in many meaningful and lasting ways. And these changes in living style often come about rather quickly. This makes sense; the Type A does everything intensely, including learning to be less intense. So, too, with couples who organize around Type A reactivity. When such people decide to take seriously the task of enhancing their marital and family life, they make smoke on the tracks of progress in accomplishing this goal.

The healthy Type A partners do two basic things: (1) They implement the suggestions outlined in chapter 7 for creating marital intimacy; and (2) they use the marital process as an aid in changing Type A reactions. Most important, they approach the process of improving their health and their marriage in an open and gracious manner. They honestly and caringly identify Type A patterns, and they use the nurturing environment of their family and marriage to help each other learn to be more comfortable in efforts to reprogram old Type A reaction habits. They cooperate rather than struggle or compete with each other in this regard.

The marriage then becomes a place of increasing intimacy. Such couples provide each other with a place of trust and emotional refuge as they work together to overcome Type A patterns, using strategies like those outlined in the following chapter.

Summary

Obviously, a Type A behavior pattern can be either a source of energy or the destroyer of intimacy in a marriage. It should also be obvious that if either of you is Type A, you must work consciously to keep this coping style in check. Otherwise, this way of reacting to the world will seriously hurt your marriage.

In the following chapter, I outline various strategies that successfully control the effect of Type A patterns on marriages. I also outline many strategies that researchers have found effective for individuals who want to modify their Type A style. This list of strategies is no more exhaustive than the energy level of a Type A reactor is exhaustible. I have learned to respect, appreciate, and admire the endless energy and creativity of Type A individuals and couples who decide to use their good stuff to make their marriages better. I hope that the following pages will simply stimulate your own creative processes.

Twelve

Strategies for Changing Type A Patterns

. . . . . .

*B*efore you can begin changing Type A reactivity, you have to answer three questions. The first question is whether changing is really necessary. Second is whether changing is even possible for a Type A individual. The last is whether you are really willing to commit to changing.

Why change? Ask your spouse, your family, or your doctor. If their reactions are not convincing, remember these two documented facts: (1) People who have poor social support systems are two to three times more likely to die from any cause, including heart disease, than people who have close social networks; and (2) research has clearly shown that Type A cardiac patients who undergo a comprehensive behavior modification program after a cardiovascular incident are nearly 400 percent less likely to have another cardiac event during the next three years than are Type A's who do not modify their behavior. (That's right: 400 percent.)

Is it really possible to change Type A reactivity? Without a doubt, many aspects of Type A pattern can be modified. Meyer Friedman and his associates have completed an extensive study that addressed this very question. Their research yielded the statistic just quoted, about the advisability of modifying Type A behavior to survive heart disease. These researchers studied and treated approximately one thousand

Type A heart attack patients and documented remarkable changes in multiple indicators of Type A reactivity among patients who underwent a behavior modification program. These changes were measured by objective observation of Type A behaviors, by patient self-reports on their own behavioral and emotional experiences, by standard psychological questionnaires, and by observations documented by the patients' spouses. I refer you to the summary of this research published by Friedman and Ulmer for further convincing information that Type A reactivity is indeed largely changeable.[13]

A word of caution is in order, however. Some aspects of Type A coping may not be easily modified. The extreme physiological reactivity of the hot reactor Type A pattern, for example (see chapter 10), may occur reflexively in some situations, but this is no reason to assume that you cannot drastically lessen the negative effect of such reactions on your life and your health. If you surround such physical reactions with more effective behavioral and cognitive coping strategies, then the net negative effect of that hot physiologial reaction on your health and on your quality of life will be significantly diminished.

Are you willing to commit to changing? I have worked with too many Type A's and have lived with my own Type A-ness for too long to be naive enough to try answering this question for you. We Type A's are individualistic, hardheaded, and overstressed enough to resist doing what other people tell us to do—even though their reactions do matter to us. You have to make up your own mind whether you will work seriously at changing. It is no small task, and it is not a single event that can be accomplished in a specific period of time. Changing your Type A-ness requires that you commit to a project of self-improvement that will last a lifetime.

Before proceeding—and certainly before answering this last question—it might be useful to understand the benefits of changing your behavior. Basically, changing Type A reactivity involves learning to decrease the prices that you pay for your inefficient ways of coping with day-to-day life. You do this by increasing your coping efficiency.

[13]M. Friedman and D. Ulmer, *Treating Type A Behavior and Your Heart* (New York: Alfred A. Knopf, 1984). Copyright © 1984 by MeyerFriedman. Reprinted by permission of Alfred A. Knopf, Inc., and Michael Joseph Ltd.

You must learn to become more aware of the specific parts of your overall Type A reactions—the specific behaviors, thoughts, and physical and emotional responses that make up your Type A patterns. Then you must practice being more selective in choosing which battles you want to fight using all your Type A bazookas, and which battles you can handle with less strenuous coping measures.

The goal is not to become laid back, unambitious, and uninvolved in your life. If you do that, life will seem to go on forever, even if you die young (bored to death). The goal is to learn to use your good stuff more selectively and more wisely and to change the self-defeating aspects of your Type A tendencies. In so doing, you free yourself from a behavioral pattern that is hurting you and the ones you love.

As is so nicely stated by Friedman and Ulmer (p. 165) and adapted here, this question of whether to modify your Type A-ness really is a question of whether you want a new set of freedoms—freedoms to

- overcome insecurity and regain your self-esteem;
- give and receive love;
- mature;
- restore and enrich your personality;
- overcome and replace old hurtful habits with new, life-enhancing ones;
- take pleasure in the experiences of your friends and family members;
- recall your past life frequently and with satisfaction;
- listen;
- play; and
- enjoy tranquility.

Research has proven the effectiveness of following a cognitive social learning approach in changing Type A patterns. This approach emphasizes modifying responses in four main areas: physiological reactions, environmental manipulations, thinking patterns, and behavioral choices.

Physiology

Once again (for the last time, I promise), you must accept the fact that a Type A person will always have an exaggerated central nervous system alarm reaction and an impoverished calming reaction in stressful situations. No matter how much you read, how much you discuss the need for changing, or how much you love each other, the Type A member or members of your marriage will always react physiologically to stress with Type A hyperreactivity. This does not mean you are doomed to the negative effects of such reactions. It simply means you must be realistic about the presence of this reaction factor and make sensible life-style choices as a consequence.

In dealing with this aspect of Type A reactivity, coping energies are best spent on preventive medicine. I emphasize to my Type A patients, for example, that they cannot afford to fuel their ready-to-flame hyperreactivity by ingesting stimulants such as caffeine, nicotine, and excessive amounts of simple sugars. It simply does not make sense to artificially speed up an already hyperreactive central nervous system. Simply use common sense in this regard: stop ingesting foods and chemicals that complicate your problem. Simple as this suggestion is, implementing it is quite difficult for most Type A's, because Type A's commonly stoke their fires before and during each day of battle by ingesting stimulants. This sets up the first leg of a two-legged physiological process. The second leg is resorting to some form of sedative in the evenings, usually alcohol or excessive eating, to slow down. Many Type A's also use prescription or over-the-counter sedatives to counter the hyperreactivity that has been elevated by the day's stresses and by their own poor choices about what they have put into their bodies.

A much more effective and obviously healthier way to calm central nervous system reactions is through regular aerobic exercise. (The value of regular exercise is emphasized in the discussion of overall stress management techniques in chapter 13.) Research has shown that aerobic exercise (exercise that elevates heart rate and breathing rate to "training" levels and keeps them elevated for twenty to thirty minutes) results in the release of naturally sedating neurochemicals called *endorphins*. In addition, regularly exercising affords a Type A person much-needed release of muscular tensions and distraction from the often grueling schedule of the day's events.

I recommend that you think of exercising as a diabetic thinks about taking insulin; it is simply something that has to be worked into the day's schedule. It is not an option, it is a physiological necessity. In choosing how to exercise, I also strongly encourage you to choose to nurture yourself. Avoid the Type A trap of turning everything, including exercise, into grueling work or a contest to be won.

It is important to have a variety of kinds of exercise available. Allow yourself to choose what to do depending on what strikes you as both an effective, safe exercise and an enjoyable way to spend an hour or so. Exercising should stir memories of the feelings you had at recess during a childhood day at school. Recess is a time to relax and move your body playfully. Your life is already too cluttered with tasks and responsibilities. Let exercising be a break from the drudgery. Maybe it would be fun to take a brisk walk around a new neighborhood one day, swim another day, and ride a stationary bicycle the next day. Avoid uncomfortably competitive forms of exercise. Relax, pace yourself sensibly, let your imagination flow in pleasurable directions, and enjoy the refreshing feeling of becoming healthier and calmer with each exercise session.

One final word about exercise: It is imperative that you consult your cardiologist about the most sensible and safe pacing in choosing an exercise program. Do not turn this into a Type A quest for creating a speedy outcome. To do so could actually hurt rather than help you.

Learning a relaxation procedure is another essential ingredient in calming reflexive physiological stress reactions. (See chapter 13 for more information on relaxation techniques.) This is particularly important for Type A personalities for—reasons that I promised not to mention again. I have noticed an interesting pattern in my own Type A patients. They invariably are able to learn a very effective relaxation strategy during their course of treatment. In fact, they usually comment on how refreshing and calming it feels to slow down and wash away muscular and psychological tensions in this manner. Many such patients actually say with amazement that they have never before experienced such soothing relaxation.

The remarkable thing is how few of them actually continue to give themselves this very available gift of relaxing once their formal treatment ceases. Relief is immediately available, but they refuse to take it. The refusal is usually justified with the lament that there is not enough time in the day to do all of one's tasks and still find time to do a relaxation exercise. Give me a break! I don't care how much of a Superperson you are, the world will survive if you take a few two-minute breaks during the day.

Remember to relax during the many breaks that occur naturally in your day's activities: waiting for a stoplight, waiting for an elevator, waiting for traffic, waiting for a spouse, or just plain waiting. If you are Type A, you have two choices in these situations: allowing tension to escalate, or simply relaxing. Learning to use such situations as cues for using your relaxation technique is a nice way to change what might otherwise be a stressor into a calming break.

It is also particularly important for a Type A person to willfully create other pauses in activity throughout the day. Periodically, take a few minutes to relax and clear your mind before moving on to your next project. Give your spouse a call just to touch base and express your affection for him or her during a busy day. Doing so not only gives your body (especially your heart) a healing moment of relief but also improves your concentration, your effectiveness in the next task, and your overall ability to manage the next stressor that comes up. It also improves your patience in reacting to each other.

As you can see, the general strategy that I recommend for dealing with the physiological aspect of Type A reactivity is to surround it with physiologically calming choices. Remember, if your Type A overreaction occurs in a context of relatively low physical and emotional tension to begin with, then the net effect of the reaction will be less damaging to you.

Environmental Factors

Type A people are notorious for not noticing pleasing aspects of their environments. This characteristic certainly leads to many lost opportunities to enhance daily life. By driving to work in a tunnel of stress-generating thoughts, for example, they miss noticing the landscape along the way or the pleasant song on the car radio. Many pleasurable feelings that could come from a moment of relishing the beauty of home or family are lost in Type A flurries of activity or thinking.

Such experiences are unfortunate and unnecessary. Noticing your surroundings is a matter of mental discipline; it does not occur naturally for Type A's. Force yourself to pause and notice. Meyer Friedman and his colleagues include in their treatment program for Type A's the homework of attending art galleries and other cultural events to exercise this capability for pausing long enough to notice. My recommendation is to begin developing this soothing and life-enriching capability at home. Notice something new about your spouse every day. Comment on what you notice in a complimentary way: "I was noticing how your eyes sparkle when you smile." " It means a lot to me that you think to turn on the outside light when I get home after dark; it makes me feel warm and welcomed by you."

Use these same observational abilities to connect more nurturingly with other family members: "I was just thinking as we were watching the kids playing; your little girl reminds me so much of you when you were that age." "I've been noticing what a wonderful father you are. You have such a loving and gentle way of responding to your kids, even when they need to be disciplined. I admire you for that."

Maybe it is difficult for you to imagine speaking such words to your loved ones. How interesting, that you would probably not hesitate to risk your own life to ensure the physical safety of your spouse or children, but you may be a coward about taking a little emotional risk to make them feel more emotionally safe and secure.

Another aspect of changing Type A reactions has to do with changing the undesirable environmental factors that you notice, once you begin noticing. Type A's discount the effect of the environment on tension and mood, but environmental factors either soothe us or stress us, whether we notice them or not. Research has shown, for example, that noise and crowding increase muscular tension and blood pressure levels, even if the respondents are not aware of the increases. It is important to provide yourself with relief from stress-generating environments. Create environments that are soothing in sight and in decibel level. A cleared desk generates less alarm reaction than a desk cluttered with reminders of all that has to be done next. Turning off radios and televisions as you chat with each other not only improves your overall communication but also may lower your tension and blood pressure levels. I refer you again to chapter 13 for other suggestions regarding management of this stress factor.

Thinking Patterns

Most Type A people spend most of their time thinking themselves into distress. In chapter 14, I discuss at length the various ways in which thinking affects emotional reactions and the ways in which we tend to engage in stress-generating thought distortions during times of alarm.

Here, I simply want to mention that an unfortunate part of Type A pattern is the tendency to think in stress-generating ways. It would be quite helpful if Type A people could hear a tape of their thinking during a twenty-four-hour period. Hearing what they say to themselves would explain much about why they react to situations and to people as they do.

Such taping of thoughts is, of course, impossible. But a good alternative is to keep a "thinking journal." Accurate and honest self-observation of the sort that comes with keeping a log of thinking patterns often results in a surprising self-revelation to Type A's. Try keeping a small notebook in your pocket, and jot down your thoughts whenever you notice yourself feeling angry, urgent, anxious, stressed, competitive, and so on. In this journal, note the situation, your feelings, your thoughts, your behaviors, and the stimuli "causing" your feelings. A typical entry in such a thinking log might read:

"Situation: Waiting for my wife to meet me for lunch.

"Feelings: Irritation, anger, frustration, hostility toward her.

"Stimuli: She's late! I keep checking my watch to document just how late she is. Also drinking coffee and smoking a cigarette to fill the time, while reading my business mail and glancing over the newspaper.

"Thoughts: She's *always* late! She was late the last time we met for lunch, too. She's probably talking on that damned phone to her stupid sister. She always chooses her family over me. I'm going to be late for my next appointment because she doesn't care enough to get here on time.

"Behaviors: Tapping fingers, shaking foot and leg. Drinking more coffee, smoking more cigarettes. Responding to the waitress in a curt, demanding manner."

What immediately becomes apparent from such a journal is the tendency to think in hostile, time-urgent, competitive ways. This tendency is inevitable for a Type A personality, but the habit is changeable. What is helpful here is identifying the ways you are thinking yourself into a Type A flurry. Then counter these thoughts with more charitable and reasonable statements.

Reason with yourself: "So she's late. I'll just take these few minutes to relax and enjoy reading the newspaper. I'll surprise her when she gets here by being calm and lovingly concerned instead of hostile. Everyone makes mistakes sometimes. I love her and I'll forgive her for this one."

Friedman and his colleagues recommend that you reexamine the broad beliefs that underlie these thinking habits. When they are stated aloud, their extremity is obvious. Work to change your self-statements in ways that remind you to slow down and take control of your behavior and of your emotions.

Type A belief: "My success is due only to the fact that I cram so much into every little space of time."

The truth: "Being in such a hurry just makes me irritable and not nice to be around. I should be proud of my ability to work hard, but my success is also due to my many talents and capabilities. I can be successful without cramming my days to overflowing."

Type A belief: "A certain amount of hostility gives me the competitive edge I need to get ahead in the world."

The truth: "My hostility is my worst cardiac risk factor. It will ruin my health and my relationships if I don't control it. I can achieve without being angry. I can motivate myself without feeling competitive with others."

Type A belief: "Other people are incompetent."

The truth: "My need to control others is fueled by my own insecurities. I need to learn to be more flexible in responding to others. So what if they don't do it my way? Even if they make a mistake, the world won't end. I need to learn to be more humble and to learn from others. It's not worth killing myself or a good relationship just because someone does something differently than I would."

Type A belief: "Showing love and kindness is a sign of weakness."
The truth: "I haven't yet learned to feel comfortable showing love and kindness. This is something worth learning to do. I have to find the courage to change, even if doing so feels uncomfortable at first."

Examples of ways to talk more sensibly to yourself about the attitudes that shape your behavior could fill an entire volume. The point is to be clear and honest in your self-appraisal and to counter any extremist beliefs or thoughts with calming and realistic self-talk.

If reasoning with yourself does not quiet these distress-producing thoughts, then simply *tell them to stop!* This method is a behavior modification technique called *thought stopping.* The thought-stopping approach to quieting negative self-talk has been particularly recommended by Redford Williams in his work with hostile Type A reactions. If you find yourself obsessively ruminating on some distress-generating thought, yell "Stop!" as loud as you can—either out loud (if the situation allows), or silently to yourself. You will be surprised at how well this little technique works to halt Type A cognitive patterns and to remind you to replace them with more soothing ways of thinking.

Finally, you may be able to stop competitive, hostile thoughts and feelings by simply placing yourself in the situation of the person or people who are causing these thoughts. Friedman and Ulmer recommend that you ask yourself these questions when you feel stuck in hostile thoughts about another person:

- What is this person's background, and what possible circumstances may have led to this sort of behavior?

- How would I feel or act if I were in this person's position, given this person's pressures, capacities, and expectations?

- How long has it been since someone caressed this person and said, "Well done. I'm proud of you"?

- Has my own initial response to this person been gracious?

- If I do become irritated or angry at this person, whom do I benefit? What do I accomplish? (pp. 219–20).

In many ways, controlling Type A thinking involves learning to think in more forgiving and tolerant ways. This is a do-able task, and it is definitely a task worth doing.

Behaviors

Changing Type A behaviors involves implementing three strategies: blocking the behaviors that are to be changed; forcing yourself to become familiar with other behaviors that are incompatible with the behaviors to be changed; and preparing for upcoming high-risk situations by rehearsing the new, more desirable behavioral responses. This model of changing can apply to any behavior pattern, but a Type A person should use these strategies particularly in changing tendencies involving hurrying, hostile or competitive reactions, and general abruptness or lack of attention in relating to others.

The rest of this section is a compilation of specific pieces of expert advice for modifying Type A behavior patterns. Much of it is my modification of the works of Meyer Friedman, Ray Rosenman, Diane Ulmer, and Redford Williams.[14] I highly recommend these works to anyone interested in more exhaustive discussion of the Type A behavioral pattern.

To change hurriedness

Increase your awareness of your here and now by taking time to recall the events of the day and of your past.

Visit museums, art galleries, or other exhibits and concentrate on noticing what you see.

Write a letter to someone describing what you saw on your outing, or just saying hello.

Show interest in others by acknowledging them, listening to them, and following up in future conversations on what was spoken about during your last talk.

[14]R. Williams, *The Trusting Heart: Great News about Type A Behavior* (New York: Time Books, © 1989), with permission. M. Friedman and R. Rosenman, *Type A Behavior and Your Heart* (New York: Alfred A. Knopf, 1974). Friedman and Ulmer, *Treating Type A Behavior and Your Heart.*

Ask a friend to a nonworking lunch and linger for a while after the meal is finished.

Spend time behaving in ways that reflect an attitude of valuing qualities worth *being* (for example, affectionate, caring, healthy), not just things worth *doing.*

Develop and participate in rituals that give you a sense of connection with a nurturing, higher order presence in life.

Take more time to complete the same amount of work you would usually rush to complete in less time.

Do and think only one thing at a time.

Even when others are moving or working slower than you like, let them complete their tasks without interruption or advice from you.

Limit your behavioral choices to things that will make a difference in your life five years from now.

Delegate tasks to others as much as possible.

Use your money to buy time by paying others to perform tasks that you do not enjoy or have to complete personally.

Read books and magazine articles that have nothing to do with your work or your major areas of worry.

Interrupt long periods of work with relaxing breaks.

Drive in the slow lane.

Listen to the end of a song on the car radio after you arrive at your destination and before you get out of the car.

Notice and comment on beauty.

Sit and do nothing for fifteen minutes.

To change hostile and competitive reactions

Learn the difference between being assertive and being aggressive. (You may want to read *A Guide to Assertive Living: Your Perfect Right,* by Alberti and Emmons.)[15]

Stop using obscenities when speaking.

When you play games with family or friends, lose on purpose and enjoy the look of accomplishment and satisfaction on the winner's face.

Smile at others, even at strangers.

---

[15]R. Alberti and M. Emmons, *A Guide to Assertive Living: Your Perfect Right* (San Luis Obispo, Calif.: Impact Publishers, 1982).

Learn to laugh at yourself when you are in the midst of a Type A flurry.

Record in your journal the things that make you angry, and take the risk of sharing this information with someone you trust.

Make restitution to those you have hurt with your hostile and competitive reactions. Simply apologize and own your responsibility for your past behavior while claiming your intention to change in needed ways.

Announce to your family your plan to develop more gracious reactions, even when you are stressed, and ask for their support and patience in these efforts.

Avoid associating with people who particularly stir your hostile or competitive feelings.

Look at yourself in the mirror periodically throughout the day to see if your face reflects irritability, hostility, or impatience.

Greet others in pleasant and cheerful ways.

Make a point of saying, "Maybe I'm wrong" at least twice a day, even when you are not certain you have made a mistake.

Apologize when conflict does occur, understanding that saying, "I'm sorry" is not the same as saying, "I'm to blame."

Do not argue with others when you know it would be pointless.

Do not strike out immediately when you feel anger toward someone. Cool down, collect your thoughts, and clarify your own position and feelings. Then, and only then, approach the other person about your concerns.

To improve your relationships

Record an hour of your conversation at home. Then listen to the tape and note any tendencies on your part to hurry others, finish their sentences for them, interrupt their speaking, or abruptly change topics without respecting their train of conversation.

Listen when others speak, and reflect back to them what you heard before you give your response to what was said.

Do not tell others what they should think and feel.

Remind yourself that people are different and that everyone is entitled to his or her own way of being.

Make note of two things that you appreciate about each of your family members every day, and tell them.

Never let a day end without expressing affection to your loved ones, both physically and verbally.

Surprise your spouse often with a small gift, a sentimental card, or a night out.

Discuss your own insecurities and fears as well as your accomplishments and talents with those you trust.

Compliment others on their ideas and accomplishments.

Let others know that you have thought or heard nice things about them.

Express appreciation to people throughout the day—to strangers who hold a door for you, to waiters, to secretaries, to family members.

Be a role model for humane reactions to other people.

Summary

Living with your own or your mate's Type A-ness is difficult, and changing your mutual reactions to these patterns is even more difficult. But the rewards of such change far outweigh the costs of the efforts. Remember to approach this aspect of your cardiac rehabilitation process with patience and common sense. No one changes easily or quickly. Be nurturing of yourselves and of each other as you address this important set of challenges. Motivate yourselves in this task with the awareness that changing Type A reactivity will not only improve your quality of life, it will also probably increase your length of life. Listen to Redford Williams:

> Research has already shown that if heart attack victims can learn to trust others and curb their free-floating hostility and angry reactions, their risk of suffering another heart attack is reduced. While harder to prove, it is likely that the benefits of such changes can be even greater for those who have not yet suffered heart damage: It is far easier to patch a small hole in the dike than it is to stem the flood once a break occurs (p. 11).

What better place to begin learning to have a more trusting and loving heart than in your own family relationships? Learning to be more caring of each other is the greatest gift you can give in your marriage. Another gift is willingness to take more appropriate care of yourself—the topic of the next chapter.

Part IV

· · · · · · ·

More than Surviving: Thriving

Thirteen

Helping Each Other by Helping Yourself

■ ■ ■ ■ ■ ■

We all know that stress reactions can be harmful to our general health, both physical and emotional. Overstressed people get sick more often and have more difficulty recovering from illness. Overstressed people can also be more difficult to live with because of their increased irritability, drivenness, fatigue, depression, anger, rigidity, or emotional uninvolvement.

Because the physical stress response directly affects the cardiovascular system, there is no doubt that stress reactions can complicate the physical course of heart illness. For everyone, not just Type A personalities, the stress response involves a temporary elevation of blood pressure: emotional alarm spurs a burst of adrenaline, which leads to increased heart rate, increased blood volume, and constriction of the peripheral vascular system.

Furthermore, when stressed, our bodies undergo a wide range of other physical changes in preparation for dealing with the stressor at hand. If not adequately soothed, these emotionally triggered physical alarm reactions can create physical illness or seriously complicate the course and degree of existing illness. Some researchers have even suggested that the prolonged physical assault of mismanaged stress can break down the immune system, thereby seriously increasing susceptibility to major illnesses and compromising the body's ability to recover from illness.

As I have already discussed, stress runs rampant throughout families that are dealing with an ill member. Even if these family members have healthy hearts, they are only human, and every human being is susceptible to the negative physical effects of uncontrolled stress. The illnesses that have been found to be caused by or complicated by stress include diabetes, inflammatory joint disease, gastrointestinal disturbances, headaches, dermatological problems, genitourinary problems, and cancer. Obviously, both heart patients and their spouses need to learn to manage stress effectively if they are to thrive.

The consequences of mismanaged stress in our daily lives are even more immediately obvious for our emotions and our relationships.

When was the last time you and your family enjoyed a week of evenly paced activities that combined time spent being productive, time for pleasure, time for intimacy, time for fun, and time for simply relaxing and enjoying your life? Most of us have far more to do than we have time to do. Our society is in the midst of a stress epidemic, and we are rapidly becoming more and more symptomatic in reaction to the endless stressors that fill our lives.

The serious emotional and physical consequences of mismanaging stress, combined with the fact that cardiac rehabilitation is itself a stress-generating process, heighten the need to evaluate yourself honestly and accurately from a stress management perspective. In fact, *the key to both individual and marital health in coping with illness is understanding and managing the stress of rehabilitation.* Individuals who manage stress better live longer. Couples who manage stress better live together more happily.

On an individual level, psychological reactions to heart disease are determined by two factors: (1) The degree of stress experienced in reaction to any stressor, including the stress of illness, varies from individual to individual; and (2) regardless of the degree of stress being experienced, different individuals vary tremendously in their style and effectiveness in managing emotional reactions. These factors combine in determining whether a given individual reacts to illness with a spirit of challenge and stimulated interest in recovery, or with moping and depressive bitterness of the sort that interferes with recovery.

Copers attend to the additional tasks brought to their lives by illness without losing overall balance in their styles of living and without letting their personality-based styles of coping lead them into any extreme behavior patterns. Mopers, on the other hand, lose their balance, both in their style of living and in their off-base attempts to calm the fears and struggles that are an integral part of the rehabilitation process. They overreact to their fears of illness in ways that make their recovery that much more difficult.

The following pages clarify how individuals can manage the stress of illness by creating a healthy balance of life activities and by understanding and controlling thoughts and behaviors. Remember to use these concepts in conjunction with what you know about personality-based coping patterns from chapters 9 and 12. Also recall the characteristics of healthy marriages as you read on.

Use these concepts as lenses through which you view both your own and your partner's reactions to the stresses that face you. In this way, you can help each other as you help yourselves to manage the effect that heart illness is having on your marriage.

Making Time for Getting Better

Getting sick is never a convenient occurrence, but for some people, illness occurs at a relatively stress-free time of life. For them, wholehearted attention and enthusiasm in responding to rehabilitation challenges are often easily summoned. One seventy-one-year-old man and his spouse, both of whom were remarkably cheerful and consistent participants in our cardiac rehabilitation program, explained their enthusiasm this way: "This heart attack has given us a new project; we were getting bored with retirement, anyway." Such a positive attitude obviously enhances overall adjustment. This couple viewed the dietary, exercise, and various life-style changes that faced them as welcome opportunities to learn about and share a new hobby.

Most of us, however, are living lives so full of commitments, responsibilities, and stress that there is no room for old hobbies, much less for the new "hobby" of cardiac rehabilitation. Creating time for, and a positive attitude toward, the rehabilitation process is much more difficult in such a psychological setting. The case study of Audie is a good example.

Audie was a fifty-six-year-old insurance agent who had run his own agency for the past eight years. He suffered a serious heart attack at the age of fifty-four, shortly after his third child graduated from high school.

Audie participated in a formal cardiac rehabilitation program religiously for the first four months after his hospitalization, but his attention to it dwindled progressively over the next year. On the request of his frustrated and fearful wife, Audie came to see me. His wife was hoping I could motivate him to participate actively in his recovery program again. His comments echoed the plight of many patients faced with this complex dilemma.

"Not motivated? Let me tell you, no one is more motivated to recover from this thing than I am. The problem is that I'm also motivated to educate my children, all three of whom are still in college; to stay afloat in my business, which is still recovering from my absences during the first year after my heart attack; and to spend some sort of time with my wife, who's had a hard enough time coping with my illness and with the kids all growing up. I'll just skip the other stuff, like my motivation to get back into my involvements in my community and back into my golf game.

"When I first had my heart attack, I was so scared that I didn't notice much except that I felt some sort of magical relief when I went to the cardiac rehab program three times a week. I kept telling myself that as long as I could get through another day taking care to eat right, rest a lot, and so on, then I'd be okay. But now I notice that life goes on. Bills still have to be paid, everyone else's needs still have to be met. Where am I supposed to get the time to do all this and still organize my life around all these new rehabilitation procedures? My life was overflowing with responsibilities to start with. I don't have time for this. It's not that I'm not motivated; I just don't have enough time."

Audie's lament is a haunting refrain in the minds of most individuals coping with illness. We live lives filled with too much to do and we have too little time to do it all.

A Balanced Life

No life event, not even a heart attack, changes the reality that we all live within the great constraint of a week that is composed of 168 hours. That's it; seven twenty-four-hour days. Within this humblingly brief amount of time, most of us are scrambling to keep four arenas alive and thriving: our self-focused involvements, such as our spirituality, personal health practices, and recreational activities; our life-work; our family and friendship relationships; and our most intimate relationship, marriage.

SELF   WORK   FAMILY   MARRIAGE

If any one of these arenas consumes too large a share of our time, some other arenas suffer. If we consistently allow involvement in one of these arenas to shrink, we become symptomatic in that arena. *There are no exceptions to this psychological rule.*

This is an important concept for understanding different psychological reactions to physical illness. At the onset of the illness, most people's involvement in some important life arena is already shrinking to the point where symptoms of neglect have developed in it. The overload of time and energy required by cardiac rehabilitation exaggerates the existing imbalance. For others, the emotional and time demands that are an inevitable part of reacting to illness create a new form of imbalance, which results in problems in personal relations or work. In either case, excessive stress is generated and experienced in reaction to illness.

For example, many heart patients have already been working excessively when heart disease is diagnosed. If such people react to heart illness by increasing their work hours or work load, they risk impairing their recovery. They may also increase the odds of experiencing family or marital problems from neglect of these arenas.

self   WORK   family   marriage

Or (another example) a grown son or daughter may react to the shock of a parent's illness with such excessive focus on the parent that his or her own life is put on hold for too long. Tensions and neglect in the other important life arenas might result in marital, work, or personal health problems for that individual, thereby furthering the stress-filled process that is already affecting the family.

self   work   FAMILY   marriage

Or, most often, the mate of a heart patient may be assigned, and assume, an unfair burden of responsibility in an effort to fulfill the role of caretaker in the marriage and in family life. Many people already live with this overload of responsibility for soothing the feelings of everyone else in the family. After heart illness strikes, the role of family caretaker mushrooms for cardiac spouses. They may consider withdrawing from fulfilling careers in order to be more available to oversee the rehabilitation process for other family members.

This might be a healthy choice for some people, but for others, such a change just results in unhappiness and stress. The needed balance of their life energies across the four important areas becomes seriously slanted in the directions of family and marriage at the expense of self and work.

self   work   FAMILY   MARRIAGE

This happens unless the cardiac spouse takes his or her own needs seriously enough to be assertive in negotiating a balance between caring for others and caring for self. In *Heartmates: A Survival Guide for the Cardiac Spouse*, Rhoda Levin describes her own struggle to maintain balance in her life following her husband's illness:

> One of the hardest lessons I learned as a cardiac spouse was the importance of going on with my own life. I had to alter my work schedule to account for the changes that were happening in my personal life. . . . There were days when I felt guilty for being healthy, going off to work, and leaving [my husband] at home alone. I felt uncomfortable sharing my enthusiasm and sense of accomplishment about work because I thought [my husband] might feel envious or anxious

about his own career. At other times, work was a refuge, a place where I didn't think about myself and I could focus on someone else. I needed to return to my work because it gave me stability and a sense of normalcy. It also helped to reduce my anxiety about our finances.[16]

If you are a cardiac spouse, take seriously your needs for enjoying life. Being miserable will not help you, and it will not help your mate's rehabilitation. If you are a heart patient, be sensitive to the fact that your spouse needs to live a full life in order to endure the stresses of rehabilitation. Encourage your spouse to take care of himself or herself. View your mate's continued involvement in the many important aspects of life as what he or she needs to do to remain healthy and helpful in living your life together.

A key rule in minimizing the degree of stress experienced in reacting to illness is this: *Create and maintain a reasonable balance across the major arenas of your life involvements—self, work, family, and marriage.*

Different aspects of your life naturally require more of your attention at different times of your life. However, there is no denying that you must create time enough for a reasonable degree of balance among these important areas, or some aspect of your life will become symptomatic.

Now that this new factor of illness has forced its way into your life, which of the four arenas—self, work, family, or marriage—is most important to attend to in lessening the stress of coping with rehabilitation? That is like asking which is the most important leg on a four-legged chair. Each is necessary and no one aspect is sufficient in promoting overall wellness. If reasonable balance does not exist, the whole mechanism gets off center.

Throughout the preceding paragraphs, I have emphasized the word *reasonable*. It is impossible to attain perfect balance of involvements in life. Indeed, it is impossible to attain perfection in any form. Quests for perfection only guarantee demoralizing frustration with oneself and with each other. Rather, the point here is twofold: You must learn to value the importance of all your major life arenas at the

---

[16]R. Levin, *Heartmates: A Survival Guide for the Cardiac Spouse* (New York: Pocket Books, © 1987). Reprinted by permission of Prentice Hall Press, a division of Simon & Schuster, New York, N.Y.

same time, and to appreciate "good enough" effort from self and from each other as you cope with your daily life together.

Don't blame or shame if you learn that neglect has shrunken one of your important life arenas. As the contemporary philosopher Matthew Fox says, seeing each other's imperfections allows us to feel safe enough to love and to be vulnerable to each other.[17] *Do* use the crisis of illness as an opportunity to take an honest and realistic look at how you are living, individually and together. Question yourselves and each other, "What do we need to change in order to live more fully as we are attempting to avoid death?"

Bernie S. Siegel is a surgeon who has written a wonderful book about the importance of maintaining hope in coping with chronic illness. In *Peace, Love, and Healing—Bodymind Communication and the Path to Self-Healing: An Exploration,* he states, "The great lesson people learn from life-threatening illness is the difference between what is and is not important."[18] If you react to illness by becoming more authentic in your way of living life—behaving more in harmony with what you really think, feel, need, and want—you will live more happily and, according to Siegel, you will live longer, too.

Use your illness to redirect your life and your relationship. If your realize that some important aspect of your life is being neglected in the weekly flow of your activities, help each other make room in your life to bolster the needed areas. A reasonably balanced life can withstand more stress than one that is already wobbling from imbalance.

Stress Reduction Universals

Regardless of the degree of stress you are experiencing, your style of emotional management ultimately determines the effect stress has on your overall quality of life. Notice that I use the term *emotional management* rather than the typical term *stress management*. In my opinion, the much-publicized stress management approaches have limited effec-

[17]M. Fox, *Original Blessing* (Santa Fe, N.Mex.: Bear & Co., 1983).

[18]B. Siegel, *Peace, Love, and Healing—Bodymind Communication and the Path to Self-Healing: An Exploration* (New York: Harper & Row, 1990), p. 89.

tiveness in soothing the stress of illness because they fail to address the thinking patterns and relationship complexities that underlie stress reactions to illness.

I elaborate on these points in the final two chapters. But first, let us briefly review in this chapter 12 major stress management strategies. Remember, these strategies are necessary, but not sufficient, to accomplish overall emotional management.

1. Getting regular *physical exercise* helps relieve emotional and physical tension. Aerobic exercise has also been found to stimulate neurochemical changes that have antianxiety and antidepressant effects. Basically, such exercise naturally soothes our nerves and elevates our sense of well-being.

2. Effective stress managers make *sensible nutritional choices*. We all have heard that we are what we eat. This adage is usually applied to our physical health, but I think the concept also applies to our emotional condition. When it comes to stress, particular nutritional culprits are sugar, caffeine, and other stimulant drugs, such as nicotine. Overstimulating the central nervous system makes relaxation impossible and sets up the likelihood of resorting next to some unhealthy form of self-sedation like overeating or usage of alcohol or other sedating drugs. Eating nutritiously and limiting intake of activating or sedating drugs, on the other hand, increase energy and promote a sense of physical and emotional stability.

3. Of special importance is the fact that many *prescribed heart medications* may have negative emotional side effects. Unwanted side effects can occur with any form of medication, but blood pressure medicines can be particularly troublesome in this regard, because these drugs work directly on the body's central nervous system. Different heart patients report a wide range of reactions to any single medication; no two people react in exactly the same way to any one drug. In addition to sexual performance problems (see chapter 8), the negative side effects of heart medicines can include fatigue, depression, confusion, nightmares, insomnia, and nervousness.

Needless to say, these reactions to medication are stressors in themselves. If you are certain that your emotional discomfort is being caused by medication and not by mismanagement of stress, consult your physician about the possibility of trying an alternate drug. If you find that you have to live with these stressful side effects, the need for taking good care of yourself in the ways described in this chapter is further underscored.

4. Implementing *time management* strategies is a necessary part of controlling overall stress levels. Getting more organized about your life involvements, prioritizing your daily activities, and sticking with the task at hand by minimizing time-wasting interruptions are all useful components of effective time management.

5. Adapting a *slower pace of life* is surprisingly effective in lessening day-to-day stress. Pausing for a few moments between tasks simply to relax or to engage in some pleasurable activity has the effect of disrupting the gradual buildup of stress and tension that inevitably occurs as the day progresses.

6. Stress is also lessened by employing commonsense strategies to control the amount of noise and other negative *environmental stimuli* we face each day. We relax more easily if we are in quiet, spacious, aesthetically pleasing spaces. In contrast, physical indicators of stress such as blood pressure and muscular tension levels elevate in response to noise or space crowding. In this vein it is important, for example, to turn the car radio to the soothing music station while you are driving (or perhaps turn it off). Or to make it a priority to spend part of each day alone in your favorite part of your home or community, taking time to slow down, center your energies, and clear your mind.

At this juncture in an emotion management seminar that I recently taught, a man raised his hand and protested, "I have a relaxing place like that where I unwind, but I still have high blood pressure." When I asked him where this quiet place was, he replied, "Bermuda." I asked him when he had last visited Bermuda, and he said five years ago. "When are you planning to return there?" I asked. "When I retire," he said. This man did not realize that so far, at least, he had relaxed only once in his entire life.

The point, of course, is to create and use de-stressing environments in *daily* living. Vacations are fun, but they occur too infrequently to be of any major help in managing daily stress in most of our lives.

7. Effective stress managers limit the number of *life transitions* they

face within a given period of time, if possible. Any major life change requires adjustments and is therefore stress generating. In a major research study conducted by Thomas Holmes and Richard Rahe, heart patients were found to have undergone more major life transitions in the several years preceding their illness than a comparable group of individuals who did not develop heart disease.[19] Most interesting, the researchers found that the stress-generating changes in many of their patients' lives were joyful events: job promotion, birth of a new family member, marriage, purchase of a new home, and so on. Of course, many others experienced negative transitions such as job loss, death of a loved one, and divorce.

The point is that any major life change is stressful, because change requires that you adjust or adapt. Controlling stress means limiting the number of major changes you must deal with at one time, if possible. For example, each year I am consulted by a number of people seeking support for their decisions to turn down some positive opportunity, such as a job promotion, simply because accepting the opportunity would push them into stress overload. Choosing not to create unnecessary additional stress during a high-transition period of life is always wise.

For others, such as you who are coping with the multiple changes that accompany illness, managing major life changes involves (1) recognizing and accepting the seriousness and inevitability of this kind of stress and (2) countering the elevation of stress that comes with all these changes by engaging in the various stress and emotional management strategies discussed here. If you are in a situation of forced multiple transitions, you must be more careful to make healthy stress-managing choices in your daily life.

8. Researcher Ethel Roskies emphasizes that one of the most effective antidotes to stress is *pleasure*.[20] Unfortunately, many of us mistake aversion relief for pleasure. The relief you feel when you finally get some dread task over with, or when you finally work your way to the

[19]T.H. Holmes and R.H. Rahe, The social adjustment rating scale. *Psychosomatic Research* 11 (1967): 213–18.

[20]E. Roskies, *Stress Management for the Healthy Type A: Theory and Practice* (New York: Guilford Press, 1987).

bottom of your list of things to do, is certainly a positive emotional experience. But this relief is comparable to how you feel when you get rid of a headache: being out of pain feels better than being in pain, but not having a headache does not necessarily mean you are feeling great; it just means that having a headache feels worse. So, too, with stress and pleasure. Completing stress-generating tasks is not the same as engaging in truly pleasurable activities. Effective stress managers incorporate joyful experiences into their lives.

What activities make you laugh and tingle in anticipation? Do you know how to give yourself permission to participate in them without guilt? Do you engage in them regularly—that is, daily or weekly—for pure pleasure? Of course, this notion of pleasure is totally subjective according to an individual's likes and dislikes on a given day. It is possible to get just as excited today in anticipation of watching a movie and eating popcorn this evening as you were yesterday in anticipation of a romantic evening of pleasure with your favorite person. Effectively managing stress involves learning to identify and respond to this internal sense of what would be soothingly pleasurable on a given day. Have some fun; you will live longer.

9. Learn a *relaxation procedure* and use it daily. The physical stress response described at the beginning of this chapter occurs reflexively in reaction to any stressor. This is a real problem in our lives, because our days are filled with multiple stressors. Fortunately, a physical antidote to the stress response is available to us in the form of the relaxation response. The relaxation response is a series of physical reactions that is the biological opposite of the stress response. Our bodies cannot experience anxiety and relaxation at the same time. Herein lies an important universal guideline in managing stress: A relaxation procedure used daily reduces stress.

The relaxation response does not occur reflexively, as does the stress response. You must therefore make conscious note of the need to relax periodically throughout the day, using your favorite relaxation procedure. Here is the other key notion about relaxation: It doesn't matter what you do to achieve physical relaxation; just do it!

For some, learning a formal relaxation procedure is helpful. Such procedures are taught in numerous stress management and relaxation training books; at seminars on yoga, transcendental meditation, and other thinking-control procedures; and through such treatment procedures as biofeedback training in relaxation. Praying stimulates the relaxation response for many people. Listening to a soothing piece of music relaxes others. Engaging in some form of self-hypnotic process such as gazing at a fire in the fireplace, taking a warm bath, or daydreaming works for others. Learning to turn on the relaxation response is like learning to ride a bicycle; once you "get it" you never forget it. The more you relax, the easier it becomes to do so.

I recommend that you commit yourself for three weeks to spending one block of twenty minutes each day concentrating on using a relaxation procedure. Use your favorite form of relaxing repeatedly, or vary the procedures to avoid boredom. How you get there does not matter; just get to relaxation. If you stick to your commitment for three weeks, you will probably find you have formed the relaxation habit.

In addition—and, I think, more important—I recommend taking many mini relaxation breaks throughout the day. It is wise to take advantage of the many "waiting" breaks that occur naturally throughout the day. While waiting at a stoplight or standing in line at the grocery store, remind yourself, "Just relax." Enjoy the break rather than creating tension for yourself by noticing how slow the light or the checkout line is. Just remembering the last time you used your favorite relaxation procedure will give you at least a brief moment of the soothing relaxation. This is a very effective way to quickly disrupt the physical stress that builds up as the day progresses.

10. Two stress-reducing and physically healing tools that can be used in conjunction with the relaxation response are *cognitive rehearsal* and *positive mental imaging*. The basic concept here is that, during the state of deep relaxation, our emotions and our bodies are very responsive to suggestion.

As is discussed in the following chapter, many of our negative emotional reactions to illness are determined by negative thinking processes. In fact, most of us spend most of our days in a state of negative self-hypnosis: we repeatedly and reflexively fill our minds with self-defeating dialogue and images, and our bodies and emotions tend to cooperate with these negative self-suggestions. On the other hand, as is pointed out by authors John Grinder and Richard Bandler in their book *Trance-Formations*,[21] it is well-documented that exceptional performers of any sort use positive self-suggestion to enhance their confidence and their performance. For example, athletes perform better when they learn to image themselves winning.

A great concert pianist once stated that the key to his virtuosity was his technique of preparing for a performance by rehearsing as much mentally as physically. In fact, he said he played a piece of music over and over in his mind, visualizing his hands on the keyboard, imagining the touch of his fingers on the keys with each note, and hearing the results of these imaginary motions, until he was able to play the piece perfectly. Only then did he sit at the piano and let his body cooperate with the positive mental programming that he had created.

Day to day, effective stress managers prepare for the multiple performances that comprise life with just such positive imaging and cognitive rehearsal. Relax your body and picture yourself taking this sense of emotional control with you throughout the coming day. Mentally prepare yourself for your upcoming day by forcing yourself to picture the day's events and your reactions as comfortable and going smoothly.

If you do not train yourself to perform positive imaging, negative and self-defeating imaging will occur automatically. Just as you must consciously remember to relax physically to counter reflexive stress reactions, so, too, must you consciously remember to mentally program effective stress management expectations to ward off anxiety-generating ways of thinking.

A fascinating body of research is accumulating that suggests that meditation, positive mental imaging, and relaxation affect the body as well as the mind. This research has particularly addressed recovery from heart illness and cancer. Dean Ornish of the Preventive Medicine Research Institute in San Francisco has published extremely hopeful research on the benefits of relaxation training in treating heart illness. Ornish has shown that cholesterol levels and arterial plaque can be

---

[21]J. Grinder and R. Bandler, *Trance-Formations: Neuro-Linguistic Programming and the Structure of Hypnosis* (Moab, Utah: Real People Press, 1981).

lessened by a program of overall life-style change, diligent attention to diet management, and weekly group meetings in which relaxation methods are used.[22]

In their work at the Cancer Counseling and Research Center in Dallas, Texas, Carl and Stephanie Simonton have shown that a procedure that involves actually picturing one's body healing internally may lead to positive physical changes in the body's immune system. These researchers report remarkable results in the effectiveness of this process in controlling, and in some cases actually reversing, the course of cancer.[23]

Although no definitive research has yet been published that demonstrates similar healing effects of positive mental imaging in dealing with heart disease, modifying this technique to fit your illness is worth a try. Here is a brief sample of the kind of meditation involved in positive mental imaging:

Relax and picture healing agents in your bloodstream flowing throughout your body, dissolving bad cholesterol deposits and cleansing your cardiovascular system. Visualize your heart and lungs as strong and healthy, nurturing you with every beat and breath. With each breath, allow this picture of internal healing and cleansing to move to each adjacent internal body region, slowly and systematically. Let yourself see and feel your muscles strengthening in response to the increased exercise that you have been doing, and visualize the nutrients that are being released in your body from the healthy foods that you are eating. See yourself growing stronger and healthier each time you relax.

Many physicians believe it is very wrong to add stress to the lives of patients who are coping with a chronic illness by implying that they can cure themselves if they will only learn to manage stress better, think more positively, or use healing imaging techniques. I agree with this warning. There is no guarantee that better stress management or imaging or any other psychological techniques will actually change your cholesterol level or improve your heart's functioning. But so

[22]D. Ornish, *Dr. Dean Ornish's Program for Reversing Heart Disease* (New York: Random House, 1990).

[23]S. Simonton, *The Healing Family: The Simonton Approach for Families Facing Illness* (New York: Bantam Books, 1984). W. Simonton, S. Matthews-Simonton, and J. Creighton, *Getting Well Again* (Los Angeles: Jeremy P. Tarcher, 1978).

what? There also is no evidence that such techniques will not work. Even if such mental gymnastics do nothing but help you feel reassured, relaxed, and motivated to continue making healthy choices, then the little bit of effort involved is certainly worthwhile. I do not recommend these techniques as a challenge to you to self-heal. I simply recommend them as a tool that may help soothe you.

Think positively. Think soothingly. Think in terms of healing.

11. One of the greatest causes of stress and one of the most effective soothers of stress is *intimate interpersonal relationships*. Of course, managing intimate relationships is basically what this book is all about, so I will not belabor this point here. I simply emphasize that effective managers of stress surround themselves as much as possible with nurturing, affirming, and comfortable relationships. In addition, they avoid or eliminate from their lives people whom they experience as toxic. A toxic person is defined as anyone to whom you react with gut-wrenching discomfort, fear, anxiety, anger, apprehension, competitiveness, or insecurity. In other words, to manage stress effectively, fill your life as much as possible with comfortable relationships and weed out of your life (or change) the ones that make you feel uncomfortable.

12. In addition to attending caringly to intimate relationships, effective managers of emotion surround themselves with *social support*. This is especially important when coping with illness. Research has shown that social support of the sort that comes from family, coworkers, neighbors, friends, and religious and civic groups tends to disappear quickly after patients are discharged from the hospital.

It is important to be assertive in finding and participating in programs or relationships that give you three kinds of support: (1) emotional support that helps reduce feelings of aloneness or fears regarding your situation, (2) information that educates you about the physical and emotional tasks of rehabilitation, and (3) practical information about ways of dealing with tangible aspects of the life changes that come with cardiac rehabilitation (such as financial changes, medical procedures, career changes, and diet modifications).

In this regard, it is most helpful to join a formal cardiac rehabilitation program. Such programs are available throughout the world, and you can probably obtain information about facilities in your area simply by contacting the office of any cardiologist. Or you can call your state or national chapter of the American Heart Association, the American Lung Association, or the national offices of the American Association for Cardiovascular and Pulmonary Rehabilitation for assistance. (See appendix A for addresses and phone numbers.) If no formal cardiac rehabilitation program is conveniently available to you, tell your doctor you are interested in meeting other couples or individuals who are facing similar challenges. Soon your phone will be ringing with the opportunity to start your own cardiac couples support group.

Of course, I strongly believe it is important for spouses to be included in cardiac rehabilitation programs. Unfortunately, not all formal ones include spouses. Some areas are developing special support groups for spouses of heart patients. Help in this regard is available from the sources listed in appendix A. I readily recognize the benefits of separate support groups for heart patients and for spouses of heart patients, but I feel strongly that it is more important for heart patients and spouses to meet together in support groups that are tailored for cardiac couples. Information about Cardiac Couples, a support program that I have developed, is available from the address listed in appendix A.

Summary

All the preceding factors are essential if you are to manage your emotions positively. After all, following such holistic guidelines to healthy living only makes sense.

In order to be healthy, you must

• live life in a balanced fashion;

• take care of your body;

• control how you use your precious time and energies;

• learn to picture yourself coping and healing;

• "take care of business" in important relationships in your life; and

• establish and participate in support systems.

But, again, my point is that although these factors are necessary, they are not sufficient for managing your emotions when coping with illness. In dealing with the unique stresses of illness, you must particularly attend to your attitudes and to your philosophy as a couple.

Fourteen

The Importance
of Attitude

■ ■ ■ ■ ■ ■

*I*t is no secret that the way we think affects the way we feel. Psychologist Albert Ellis was one of the first to point out that if we control our cognitions—thinking patterns that take the form of self-talk or of pictures that we flash in our minds—we can control our emotional reactions more effectively.

For example, suppose that one day as I am leaving for the office, my wife says to me, "Your shirt doesn't match the color of your pants." I might respond to this event with a lot of bothersome thoughts based on my own insecurities: "She doesn't like the way my clothes look. She doesn't like the way I look. She's never liked my looks. She's probably running around with the next-door neighbor."

Such thinking would obviously generate a set of negative emotional reactions: anger, insecurity, and jealousy. These painful emotions would be reactions to my own thinking process, not direct reactions to my wife's comments.

On the other hand, I might respond to this same event ("Your shirt doesn't match the color of your pants") with thoughts related to a belief that my wife loves me: "It's nice that she noticed. It feels good that she cares enough and trusts me enough to tell me. This is a sign of our intimate connection." This second set of internal statements would obviously generate a very different emotional reaction: feeling soothed by being noticed and loved.

An important fact to know in controlling our emotions is that thinking patterns, just like gross motor behavioral patterns, can become habitual. In other words, if we think in certain ways often enough, we get stuck in the rut of thinking in these ways. We then get stuck in the habit of feeling the emotions that come with these ways of thinking. It is as though thinking in a certain way long enough and hard enough eventually leads to the development of an attitude that then colors our general emotional reactions.

This point is particularly important in understanding our reactions to any ongoing stressors, such as the stressor of cardiac rehabilitation. Some people develop a Born to Lose attitude; they feel doomed by the perspective that they have no choice over this matter of managing their emotions now that stress has reached seemingly unmanageable levels. Julia's attitude is an example.

Julia was a fifty-four-year-old attorney who had responded to her illness by getting bogged down in depression and who had no motivation to reenter the mainstream of her life. In discussing her illness, she made the following statements, each of which conveys the self-defeating attitude that underlay her paralysis in reacting to her illness: "All I see when I look to the future is my family and life in general going on without me. . . . I should have taken better care of myself, but I just didn't have the courage to control my own behavior. . . . It's hard to feel motivated to go on when you feel like the end just began."

Other individuals seem to follow the motto that we all are Born to Choose our emotional reactions, even when the adaptive tasks that face us are not of our choosing. Lucy's reactions are an example of this way of reacting to illness.

Lucy was a sixty-seven-year-old housewife who had suffered a severe heart attack but who had experienced minimal symptoms of emotional distress in the ensuing years of her life. Her overall attitude toward her illness and rehabilitation was obvious.

"When I got sick, my husband and I decided that this illness was a not-so-gentle warning to us to get our individual and collective acts together. We weren't living any awful life at the time, but we just weren't paying much attention to what our life and our relationship was really all about.

"While I was still in the hospital, we vowed to each other that when I came home, we would begin noticing and enjoying the little things that make up every day and that add up to a marriage. I haven't had time or reason to be depressed. In many ways, I've had better quality of life since my heart attack than I ever did before."

The differences in attitude about illness expressed by Julia and Lucy have obvious implications for the likelihood that these women will adjust differently to heart disease. They both are suffering from essentially the same illness, yet one's life is being ruined in the process while the quality of the other's marital and emotional life is actually improving during cardiac rehabilitation.

Cognitive Distortions

Unfortunately, during times of increased stress most of us, like Julia, automatically engage in thinking processes that hurt rather than help in managing the stresses of the moment. It is as though Mother Nature played a cruel trick by making us so that we naturally compound our pain during times that are already filled with pain.

Our first responses when we are faced with stressful situations almost always involve self-statements that fuel negative emotions. These stress-generating forms of thinking are referred to as *cognitive distortions*, and they vary in form. Each of these ways of thinking is guaranteed to increase worry and prolong stress.

In his book, *Feeling Good: The New Mood Therapy*, David Burns lists the most frequently occurring cognitive distortions.[24] These adjustment-squelching modes of thinking are explained in the following pages, accompanied by examples from the perspective of both a heart patient

[24]D. Burns, *Feeling Good: The New Mood Therapy* (New York: New American Library, 1980).

and a concerned family member. In addition, examples of more realistic, adaptive responses are given.

All-or-Nothing Thinking

This is perfectionistic, black-or-white thinking that involves trying to
force your experiences into absolute categories, thereby interfering
with the opportunity to be soothed by "good enough" experiences.

Distortion

HEART PATIENT: I can't find the time to exercise regularly because
my work travel disrupts my routine, so why exercise at all?

FAMILY MEMBER: He got chest pains the last time we argued. I'd
better keep my feelings to myself from now on.

Adaptive Thinking

HEART PATIENT: Any exercising is better for me than no exercising
at all.

FAMILY MEMBER: Uncontrolled arguing is stressful for all of us. We
need to learn more effective ways of communicating difficult feelings.

Overgeneralization

Here, you frighten yourself by concluding that something that happened once will occur over and over again.

Distortion

HEART PATIENT: I tried that treadmill test once, and my legs and
chest ached for days afterwards. I won't do that again.

FAMILY MEMBER: I have a friend who has a cousin whose husband
died from a heart attack during sex. We'd better just abstain.

Adaptive Thinking

HEART PATIENT: At least I have one experience of treadmill testing
under my belt. Now that I know what to expect, it won't be such a
strange experience next time.

FAMILY MEMBER: From all I've read, sex seems to be cardiovascularly safe if commonsense guidelines are followed about how and when. We'll relax and learn to make it safe and fun.

Selective Perception

This way of thinking is like using a mental filter that leads you to see only the distressing details of situations.

Distortion

HEART PATIENT: I feel terrible about myself; I ate bacon once this month, and I know I'm not supposed to.

FAMILY MEMBER: All Daddy does since his heart attack is sit in that recliner, waiting to die.

Adaptive Thinking

HEART PATIENT: I'm doing a reasonably good job of managing my diet. I've eaten bacon only once in the last thirty days.

FAMILY MEMBER: Daddy rests more frequently since his heart attack. He still does get a fair amount of exercise, though.

Discounting

This involves disqualifying the positive aspects of a situation or transforming neutral or positive experiences into negative ones.

Distortion

HEART PATIENT: The results of my medical checkup today were no better than three months ago. All this rehab business obviously isn't helping me.

FAMILY MEMBER: Since her heart attack she suddenly wants to act like we're some sort of loving family, as if all the past stuff had disappeared overnight.

Adaptive Thinking

HEART PATIENT: I wish these medical tests would show me to be improving steadily, but stabilizing is better than getting worse.

FAMILY MEMBER: I have to admit that she obviously has a different attitude about us since her heart attack. We still have problems, but maybe this is a start in the right direction.

Mind Reading

This occurs when you arbitrarily jump to a negative conclusion without checking the facts.

Distortion

HEART PATIENT: This blood pressure medicine makes me impotent and depressed. I guess I'll just have to live with that.

FAMILY MEMBER: She's quiet today. I hate it when she gets preoccupied with the fear that she won't see another Christmas.

Adaptive Thinking

HEART PATIENT: I've had sexual performance changes and I've been depressed since starting this medicine. I need to ask my doctor if this is usual and if there might be another blood pressure medicine that I can try.

FAMILY MEMBER: You seem quiet today. What's going on?

Fortune-telling

This term refers to *catastrophizing,* or imagining the worst-case scenario and then taking that dismal prediction as fact.

Distortion

HEART PATIENT: This might be the last year of productivity I have. I'd better cram in as much work as I can, while I can.

FAMILY MEMBER: First this heart attack, next it'll be forced medical retirement, then boredom and depression for the rest of our lives. I can't take this.

Adaptive Thinking

HEART PATIENT: I wonder how many years of productivity I have left. There's no way to predict, so I might as well enjoy the year at hand.

FAMILY MEMBER: I don't know what's going to come next, but we're surviving so far.

Magnification and Minimization

The distortion of magnification involves focusing on your faults, fears, and imperfections in a manner that exaggerates their importance. It is as though your flaws are being viewed through a magnifying glass. At the same time, you may minimize your strengths and assets; the soothing aspects of life seem to be viewed out of the wrong end of binoculars, thereby diminishing their positive impact.

Distortion

HEART PATIENT: My life is pretty much back to normal; big deal. I have to depend on this medicine that makes me feel washed out. Sometimes I feel like I'm just going through the motions.

FAMILY MEMBER: Her blood pressure is stable. Her diet is good. Her exercise tolerance is up. But her cholesterol is still high. She'll never recover at this rate.

Adaptive Thinking

HEART PATIENT: I hate the way this medicine makes me feel washed out, but I sure am glad my life is pretty much back to normal. This tiredness might just be the price I have to pay for enjoying the other parts of my life.

FAMILY MEMBER: I'm worried that her cholesterol is still high, but I have to give her credit; she's managing most of the risk factors wonderfully. Compared to six months ago, she's doing great, overall.

Emotional Reasoning

In this form of distorting, you take feelings as evidence of some "truth" and then make catastrophizing implications based on it.

Distortion

HEART PATIENT: My kids visited yesterday and I was too tired to even talk much with them. If I feel this way, I must not be recovering. I guess life is just going to be lonely and miserable from here on out.

FAMILY MEMBER: I'm anxious and scared silly that he's going to have another heart attack. I know my fear means that he's just not taking good enough care of himself. It makes me so angry that he doesn't care any more than that.

Adaptive Thinking

HEART PATIENT: Just because I had a "down" day yesterday doesn't mean I'll stay stuck. I had good and bad days even before my heart attack.

FAMILY MEMBER: I'm scared a lot, and I wish he could soothe my fears. Maybe it would help if I wrote down the things he *is* doing to take care of himself. If I see proof that he's trying, then I might not be so angry.

Labeling and Mislabeling

This is an extreme form of overgeneralization in which you create a negative self-image by evaluating yourself exclusively on one less-than-perfect aspect of your life or experience.

Distortion

HEART PATIENT: I'm forty-nine years old and I've already had a stroke and bypass surgery. What kind of man would let this happen to himself? I'm a failure as a husband, a father, and a person.

FAMILY MEMBER: I'm in charge of the cooking in this family, and his cholesterol is sky high. I'm a failure as a wife and mother.

Adaptive Thinking

HEART PATIENT: My health isn't so good for being as young as I am. But I've done a lot right in my life, including how I'm reacting to this illness. I'll just do the best I can, and go from there.

FAMILY MEMBER: I wish I had learned about this low-cholesterol cooking years ago, but I just didn't. Now that we're all learning about heart disease a lot is changing, including the ways I cook. At least I'm willing to do what I can to help my husband recuperate now that we understand how.

Personalization of Blame

This occurs when you unfairly assume responsibility for a negative event by blaming yourself for being the sole cause of the misfortune. The result is bittersweet. On one hand, personalization of blame momentarily soothes anxieties that come whenever you realize that you are not always in control of important things that happen to you. In blaming yourself, you indirectly create the soothing illusion that you might have been able to control what happened. On the other hand, personalizing blame usually leaves you feeling the useless pain of guilt. You need encouragement, but you shame yourself instead.

Distortion

HEART PATIENT: The only reason I'm sick now is that I'm a lazy slob. If I had taken better care of myself, this would never have happened. There's no one to blame but me.

FAMILY MEMBER: I should have known that my taking that new job was going to create too much pressure for her. Now she's had a heart attack and it's all my fault. If I had been more successful in life, she would have had an easier time of it, and this wouldn't have happened.

Adaptive Thinking

HEART PATIENT: I know I need to start taking better care of myself in a lot of ways, and I wish I had begun long ago. But no one can say for sure why one person develops heart disease and another doesn't. Just look at my brother: he eats, drinks, smokes, and stresses more than I do, and he's healthy as a horse!

FAMILY MEMBER: I truly do wish life were less stressful; maybe that would have made a difference in my wife's health. I've just done the best I could do in my life, and all I can do now is try to recuperate along with her.

It is important to understand that the distorting, maladaptive modes of thinking that have been described occur reflexively and automatically as initial responses to stressful situations. Whether you are dealing with some part of cardiac rehabilitation (for example, an upcoming checkup by the cardiologist) or with day-to-day stressors (for example, a busy day of errands), your initial response will usually be to think yourself into more stress than the situation may warrant.

I believe we have no choice in this matter. Stress-generating thinking patterns occur reflexively in reaction to stressors. However, we do have the power to choose what happens next. As psychiatrist Viktor E. Frankl stated in *Man's Search for Meaning*, his book about his experiences in World War II concentration camps, "Everything can be taken from a man but one thing: the last of the human freedoms—to choose one's attitude in any given set of circumstances, to choose one's own way."[25]

If you notice yourself getting caught up in stress-generating ways of thinking, it is possible to soothe your stress by forcing yourself into a more reality-based appraisal of the situation. Caringly reminding and helping each other to think realistically is an important part of managing emotional reactions to illness.

Learning to Think Realistically

Thinking styles are made up of habitual ways of viewing the world or of talking to yourself. You can change these habits, just as you can stop habits such as biting your fingernails. The way to change a maladaptive thinking habit is to develop realistic thinking habits.

I am not referring to the stereotypical notion that one should learn to "think positively." In my opinion, thinking positively sometimes involves attempting to lie to yourself, and such lying can actually increase stress and tension. This is especially true in a family dealing with illness. It is important to admit out loud that no one is happy about getting sick or about a loved one going through difficult times. Pretending only creates distance among family members, and it does not really help anyone feel better, anyway.

It is far better to use realistic thinking in place of the lies that are promoted in the catastrophizing, blaming, fear-generating cognitive distortions. To start learning realistic thinking, reread the examples of adaptive thinking in this chapter for suggestions on realistic ways of

[25]V. Frankl, *Man's Search for Meaning* (New York: Touchstone, 1984), p. 184.

thinking about illness and rehabilitation. Then learn to list the pros and cons of a situation realistically. Try writing them down. This exercise will help you get rid of the bad feelings that come from looking just at the cons. It also gives you the opportunity to be soothed by seeing the pros.

By learning to think realistically, you can avoid developing self-defeating attitudes that can be dangerous to your health. In a Harvard University study originated by George Vaillant and continued by Martin Seligman and Christopher Peterson, a group of nearly a hundred men were followed for forty years to evaluate the relationship between mental and physical health. The findings? Mental attitudes were clearly shown to affect both susceptibility to disease and ability to recover from illness. Specifically, these researchers found that pessimistic individuals deteriorated in health more quickly beginning around age forty-five. Furthermore, this vein of research proposes that thinking in ways that promote optimism can actually enhance your health and guard you against illness.[26]

Summary

Thinking habits help determine emotional reactions. Emotional habits affect overall health and reactions to illness. Listening to your own self-talk and also noticing the statements your partner makes can tell you much about the causes of your moods and reactions to this illness.

If you or your mate is stuck in self-defeating thinking habits, both your relationship and your rehabilitation will suffer. Your specific ways of thinking about illness can add up to a general philosophy about your overall rehabilitation process. This philosophy will either help you to heal or cause you to suffer.

[26]See C. Peterson, M. Seligman, and G. Vaillant, Pessimistic explanatory style is a risk factor for physical illness: A thirty-five-year longitudinal study, *Journal of Personality and Social Psychology* 55, 1 (1988): 23–27; and M. Seligman, *Learned Optimism* (New York: Alfred A. Knopf, 1990).

Fifteen

Healing

■ ■ ■ ■ ■

Coping with heart illness as a couple requires a wealth of information and even more love and courage. Thus far, we have examined this topic from a wide range of perspectives:

- Illness is a stressor.

- Recovery is an ongoing process, not an event.

- We differ in our reactions to the stress of illness because of individual differences in personality makeup.

- We can choose to create new coping patterns by modifying our personality-based coping strategies, attitudes, behaviors, and relationship processes.

- Families work like teams and can react to illness in ways that either help or hinder both physical and emotional rehabilitation for all members, not just for the identified heart patient.

- The key to successful family functioning is marital intimacy.

- Coping with heart illness often erodes marital intimacy in many ways, especially in the realm of sexual functioning.

- Cardiac couples should pay particular attention to concerns about Type A behavior patterns, because they may negatively affect overall relationship intimacy.

- The key to successful emotional adjustment to heart illness (and, many researchers would argue, to successful physical adjustment as well) is intimacy.

Throughout this book I have tried to keep my promise to provide many recommendations for managing your marriage rather than waiting until this final chapter to attempt to tie everything together. You should now be aware of a number of concepts and specific bits of information that can serve as useful tools as you manage the never-ending tasks involved in being married and coping with illness.

Several important points on the broadest levels of understanding do remain to be made, however, about the tasks of healing and growing in marriage. These points have to do with the values and philosophies that guide your psychological and behavioral choices and that, therefore, serve as the ultimate originators of your coping patterns.

Why Did This Happen to Us?

"Why did this happen to me? I didn't plan to have a spouse who would have a heart attack."

"Sure, I should be taking better care of myself in some ways. But I never thought I would have to face heart surgery. What did we do to deserve this?"

"How can I make sense out of this suffering?"

Such questions are inevitably asked by anyone coping with heart illness. Perhaps, if answered, these questions lead to increased strength and resolve in coping with what has been dealt to the sufferer. In an effort to find answers, many heart patients and their families turn to their belief in God. The problem with this tactic, as is so eloquently explained by Harold S. Kushner in *When Bad Things Happen to Good People*, is that many of us find it difficult to maintain faith in and to derive soothing from a God who "allows" suffering.[27]

If our faith fails to provide us with answers to these haunting *why* questions, we often compound the damage that illness has done by

[27]H. Kushner, *When Bad Things Happen to Good People* (New York: Avon Books, 1981).

hurting ourselves and each other with guilt, self-imposed loneliness, and anger—at self, at others, and at God. Some experts on the psychological impact of illness believe that unless we find a soothing meaning in our experience, we move more quickly toward death.

I am not a spiritual counselor or a clergyman of any kind. Nevertheless, like anyone working in a medical helping profession who has paid attention to experience, I am moved and humbled by the healing power of spiritual reconciliation. It is especially evident in work with individuals and families who have faced death. In being forced to acknowledge the brevity of life, people experience the need to make sense of their life from the perspective of a higher order than that of mundane, day-to-day existence. Without such an understanding of the meaning and purpose of our suffering, we settle into despair during times of struggle.

When a family member is in such despair, we usually find ourselves impotent to help ease the pain. Our pep talks seem to fall on deaf ears: "Come on, we've got a lot of living left to do. Cheer up!" But we may get no positive response to our happy words. Our well-intentioned reminders of God's wisdom or of some divine master plan seem only to alienate us from our suffering loved ones: "This is our cross to bear. God wouldn't have dealt us this hand if he didn't think we could handle it." Worse yet, some families react to the sufferers with the confusing message that they should be grateful for being forced to deal with this agony: "God must see you as a special person, one who can shoulder this pain and serve as an example to others."

Well-intentioned as these semispiritual lecturettes are, it is important to realize that they usually do not soothe; they only cause more pain to the suffering individual, and frustration in your relationship.

A healthy and helpful alternative in coping with suffering is to develop a healing philosophy as a couple. Whenever I treat partners who are coping with heart illness, I give them a copy of the seven reminders titled "Our Healing Philosophy" and ask them to read them aloud to each other regularly. (This list borrows heavily from the work of Kushner; I have tailored it to apply to heart illness.)

"Our Healing Philosophy"

1. We did not deserve this illness, but it happened.

2. Now that this illness has happened, there is some added pain in our life. We need to find a purpose in the pain of rehabilitation. Otherwise, our pain will simply feel like pointless suffering. Our pain can either make us bitter and envious of others or lead us to become more sensitive and compassionate. What we do in reaction to this illness will make the pain of rehabilitation either meaningful or empty and destructive to us an individuals and as a family.

3. As we struggle through this together, we need to allow each other and ourselves to be angry at the situation and try not to be angry at ourselves, at each other, or at our God. We need to remember that

Getting angry at ourselves makes us depressed. Being angry at other people scares them away and makes it harder for them to help us. Being angry at God erects a barrier between us and all the sustaining, comforting resources of religion that are there to help us. . . . But being angry at the situation, recognizing it as something rotten, unfair, and totally undeserved—shouting about it, denouncing it, crying over it—permits us to discharge the anger which is a part of being hurt, without making it harder for us to be helped.[28]

4. We will try to encourage each other to pray for strength, determination, and willpower to cope, and for the grace to remember what we still have instead of suffering over what we have lost.

5. We will try to live full lives until we die. We will try to show each other how to live and love despite our struggles. We will try to let this illness help heal our lives.

6. The question we still ask ourselves is *not,* "Why did this illness happen to us?" Rather, we will ask, "Now that this illness has happened, what can I do to cope, and who is available to help me?"

[28]Kushner, *When Bad Things Happen to Good People*, p. 108–9.

7. We need each other as allies in this journey. I am happy that you are here with me now.

Choosing Intimacy in Coping with Illness

Throughout this book, I emphasized my belief that you are Born to Choose when it comes to dealing with your individual stress reactions. I believe even more passionately that you have choices as a couple in determining your reactions to heart illness within your relationship. I believe that you only have two basic choices, however: your reactions to this illness will either (1) help or (2) hinder your marital intimacy.

Different phases of the cardiac rehabilitation process create different varieties of relationship crises. But on the broadest of levels, each of these relationship crises involves your struggle to stay on course in the developmental progression outlined in chapter 7. Relationship crisis tends to pull you backward, to make you regress to a less mature and less healthy way of functioning. Be aware of these pulls and persist in your cooperative efforts to help your relationship along this path of growth.

As you travel together, do not kid yourselves or each other about the realistic destination of this journey as a couple. Marriage does not involve undying security, or endless happiness, or never-ending intimacy. Healthy marriages settle into Good Enough Territory. Your mission as a couple is to be reasonably certain that you are not going backward in this journey. Your quest should be to discover how far you can go together as husband and wife.

I have found that the following brief marital exercise is tremendously helpful to couples who are attempting to stay on course in their marital journey. This exercise helps you consciously choose to create and embrace intimacy as a soothing balm to your fears or as an icing to the delicious cake that is your life together, in sickness and in health.

Getting Loved by Being More Loving

This exercise is based on a fact that underlies many of the techniques used by marital therapists to help couples change in positive ways: the best way to get your partner to behave in ways that you value is to stop waiting for your partner to change, and, instead, begin using your energies to be more loving in ways that your partner values. The following steps can help you create a renewed sense of teamwork and appreciation of each other as you live day to day.

1. Each of you should write a series of short sentences that describe your honest impressions of ways you can behave that you know from experience tend to be deeply satisfying and touching *to your partner.* Keep the list simple, and list your items in positive terms ("You like it when I tell you I think you're pretty"), rather than in negative terms ("You like it when I say that it looks like you're losing some weight, for a change"). Draw from all of your knowledge and experiences with your mate. Don't edit the list based on your differences from your partner; the point is to list what you know he or she likes, not what you like to do. For now, don't worry about whether you are willing to do any of the things on your list. This is not a contract; it's a way of reminding yourself that you know much about how to be powerfully positive in relating to your partner. For example, your list might read:

I know that it means a lot to you when

- I give you a back rub and do not make it sexual.
- I bring you a cup of coffee in the morning before you get out of bed.
- I am willing to go shopping with you.
- I am polite and talkative when your mother calls or visits.
- I ask how your day has been and listen with interest.
- I surprise you by arranging for us to get away overnight.
- I ask you to take a walk with me.
- I hold your hand when we are out with friends.

2. Next, each of you should write another list, this time cataloging those things that your partner can or does do that are especially meaningful *to you*. List things that especially touch you and leave you feeling noticed, appreciated, reassured, and loved by your spouse. Remember, be positive and descriptive, not critical. For example, this list might read:

It is very special to me when you

- Tell me I look attractive before I leave in the mornings.
- Initiate sex.
- Tell me that you think that my rehabilitation is succeeding.
- Tell me that you want to stay home on Friday night, alone with me.
- Tell me that you appreciate how hard I work and that you feel safe and protected in our life together.
- Brag to our relatives about me as a parent.
- Promise me that you will stick by me, no matter what the future brings.
- Call and ask me out to lunch.
- Make a big deal of occasions that are special to me, like my birthday, Valentine's Day, or Christmas.
- Encourage me to take time to be with my friends.
- Tell me that you admire the way I deal with my parents.

3. Next, take turns reading each other's lists. I recommend that you do this in separate rooms (or at separate times), and that you each take time to think about the important information that your partner is sharing with you in these lists. You will probably notice that some of the items listed are small things that can be done on a daily or weekly basis, while others (like taking vacations together) might be possible only occasionally.

4. Then, arrange a time to give each other your full attention, and discuss the information shared in the lists. Be caring and validating of your partner, even if some of the information in the lists makes you feel uncomfortable. Remember, you are learning how you can be a

more healing and loving partner for the person that you most love. Don't argue or debate about whether you already do the things listed, or about why your partner values the things listed on his or her list. Even if you would be uncomfortable doing some of the things listed, try to learn what is of special loving value to your spouse.

5. Based on your partner's feedback to you, both from the written lists and from your conversation, add or subtract items from your first list so that you end up with a final list that contains a concrete set of guidelines that can serve as reminders of how to be powerfully positive in dealing with your mate when you so choose.

6. Finally, agree to experiment. For a period of time (I recommend starting off with no less than two weeks and no more than one month), agree to use your best energies to be a positive source of love and healing for your mate. You do not have to promise to do all that is mentioned on your final list. Simply use this list as a reminder and as a set of guidelines about what you can do to be uniquely powerful in a loving way in your day-to-day life with your mate.

7. As the ensuing days and weeks pass, give each other feedback often regarding what you appreciate about the efforts that you see your partner making in being more loving in ways that are special to you. Do not do this with a spirit of parental monitoring; don't deliver relationship report cards to each other. Remember the point here: be positive and caring, and you increase the odds that your partner will do the same.

What do you notice as you read through this exercise? How comfortably can you create a vision of being a source of love and healing for your partner, and can you see your partner being the same for you? What interferes with this soothing way of living together? Are there aspects of your life that need to be changed so you can be more loving for each other? What do you need to begin doing more of or stop doing so much of? What do you need to forgive, forget, or simply put aside in order to be more loving partners?

Many couples need help overcoming obstacles in learning to love again. Many loving couples need help to keep their love growing.

Such help is available through marital counseling (see appendix B) and participation in couples' support group programs or marital enrichment experiences (see appendix A).

You Will Survive, But Will You Live?

Now that your life has been changed by heart illness, you must make a crucial decision, both as individuals and as a couple: What will be the meaning of your life from this point forward? Given all that you have experienced and are experiencing, all that you know of yourselves and of each other, and all that you wish for the future and lament about the past, what do you choose about your life and your marriage *starting right now*?

Your collective answer to this very important question will be the cornerstone on which your relationship will continue. Your answer to this question will shape your attitudes, your behavioral choices, your marital quality, and—I sincerely believe—your ability to cope with this illness.

Most of us clearly want a richer and more contented peace in living our lives; most of us live in quest of such contentment. But in pursuing this quest, we fail to appreciate the satisfactions that are immediately at hand. In his simple, yet extraordinary little book, *The Precious Present,* Spencer Johnson relates a profound parable of a man's lifelong intrigue with the feeling of peace and contentment that he experienced as a child whenever he conversed with a certain wise old man.[29] The story revolves around the young man's quest to obtain a precious present promised to him by the old man. The wise elder explained: "It is a present because it is a gift. . . . And it is precious because anyone who receives such a present is happy forever" (p. 9).

As the story unfolds, the young boy grows to be a man and lives in constant anticipation of the special gift. He endures repeated frustrations because he does not receive it. He searches and struggles and ponders his lack of contentment with his life. He grows ever more frustrated with the old man's failure to make a difference in his life by

[29]S. Johnson, *The Precious Present* (New York: Doubleday, 1981).

granting him the precious present. Finally, in his own middle age, and in the midst of grieving the death of the wise mentor, the man discovers that the precious gift of which the old man spoke, and which the old man modeled, is learning to live with awareness of self in the present moment.

It is unfortunate that we must often face tragedy, like the young man's loss of his beloved mentor in Johnson's parable, before we address the reality that our lives consist of the present and no more. Whether your own life and marriage were shocked by the entry of heart illness recently or long ago, the basic psychological task facing you remains the same: Learn to live each day with awareness of the choice to be happy, and learn to choose to create and enjoy the contentment and the healing that come with intimacy.

You were Born to Choose. Choose to become allies to each other, and make your present precious.

Appendix A

Resources

■ ■ ■ ■ ■

To inquire about available cardiac rehabilitation programs in your area, contact any of the following:

American Association for Cardiovascular
and Pulmonary Rehabilitation
7611 Elmwood Avenue, Suite 201
Middleton, WI 53562
(608) 831-5122

American Heart Association
7320 Greenville Avenue
Dallas, TX 75232
(214) 750-5300

American Lung Association
1740 Broadway
New York, NY 10017
(212) 315-8700

If your partner has suffered cognitive impairment from heart illness and you would like help and support in coping with his or her condition, call or write to

National Stroke Association
1420 Ogden Street
Denver, CO 80218
(303) 839-1992

For further information about support group programs designed specifically for cardiac couples or for spouses of heart patients, call or write

Cardiac Couples
c/o Wayne M. Sotile, Ph.D.
1396 Old Mill Circle
Winston-Salem, NC 27103
(919) 765-3032

The following audiocassette tapes featuring Dr. Sotile are available from the same address.

1. "Cardiac Couples: Guidelines and Exercises for Your Support Group." Advice on forming and running a support group for couples dealing with heart illness. Mini lectures that can be used to stimulate discussions on topics such as families as teams, managing the stress of rehabilitation, sex and heart illness, and others.

2. "Sexual Aspects of Cardiac Rehabilitation." The ways heart illness can interfere with sexual functioning, and specific guidelines for enhancing sexual ability and relationship intimacy. Effects of medications and aging on sexual performance, exercises to enhance relationship intimacy and sexual enjoyment, and more.

3. "In Sickness and In Health: Managing the Impact of Illness on Your Marriage and Your Family." How families work as teams and how the shock of illness can cause problems for all family members. Positive ways of dealing with both young and adult children when coping with illness.

4. "Thriving, Not Just Surviving: Cardiac Rehabilitation is More Than Just Exercise." Psychological, behavioral, and family factors that are affected by heart illness and that are

essential to healthy recovery. Understanding and controlling psychological reactions, managing your medical care, coping pitfalls to be avoided in marriage and family life, and more.

5. "Stress and Emotional Management: Keys to Healthiness." Definition, causes, and cures of stress. Self-directed exercises to pinpoint specific personality-based stress responses, ways of developing more effective emotional management habits, and more.

6. "The Couple's Journey: The Challenge of Change in Marriage." How marriages develop and how to surmount the relationship hurdles of growing and facing unexpected challenges, such as illness. Practical examples drawn from experiences of couples who thrive, keys to establishing and maintaining intimacy and passion, and more.

7. "Understanding and Living with Type A Behavior: A Guide for Couples and for Individuals." What Type A behavior pattern is and how it affects individual health as well as marriage and family life. Numerous proven strategies for changing the pattern, "confessions" of spouses of Type A's, and more.

8. "How We Differ: The Effects of Personality in Coping With Illness." Why different people react to illness in different ways, based on personality programming. A practical way to understand and change personality-based coping patterns that may interfere with adjustment.

9. "Healing Attitudes: How Do You Define 'Illness'?" The importance of attitude in recovering from illness and the difficulties faced by couples and families when those attitudes differ. Specific thinking patterns that can interfere with both spouses' reactions to illness and ways of learning more adaptive thinking habits.

10. "Men in Recovery: Sex, Intimacy and Health." How contemporary notions about masculinity can interfere with recovery. Nine "truths" about men that color their reactions

to stress, to one another, and to aspects of marriage and family life that are important in recovering from illness.

11. "Psycho-Social Aspects of Cardiac Rehabilitation: For Professionals." A model for understanding, and helping patients to cope with, cardiac rehabilitation. Illness and stress, grieving and rehabilitation, understanding personality and its effect on rehabilitation, and more.

Appendix B

Choosing a Therapist

. . . . . .

The following facts can guide you in choosing a therapist if you decide to seek general psychological or psychiatric help.

1. Different mental health professionals have different theoretical orientations. Some emphasize the need to understand and work through the pains that have resulted from past experiences and relationships, whereas others are more problem-solving and here-and-now focused in their emphasis. Choose a therapist who matches your needs.

2. Mental health therapy is provided by professionals with varying educational backgrounds. Formal education does not ensure that a given individual will be an effective therapist for you, but knowing a therapist's educational background may be helpful in your initial screening of professionals in your community.

3. Both doctoral level (Ph.D., Psy.D., and Ed.D.) and master's level (M.A., M.S., M.A.Ed.) psychologists are available. Psychologists are generally trained to help others solve their life problems and improve their ability to cope with daily living. Some do so by helping you to understand yourself better and to overcome the pain of past wounds. Others focus on teach-

ing new coping skills such as communication skills, better emotional management strategies, and relaxation techniques.

Psychologists do not prescribe medication. However, any psychologist competent enough in medical psychology to be of help to heart patients should have medical consultants available (either psychiatrists or other medical specialists) in the event that you need to be evaluated for medication.

The services of psychologists who are licensed by the state in which they practice are usually covered by general medical insurance programs. Consequently, any insurance policy that provides coverage for outpatient mental health consultation will likely help pay for the services of a licensed psychologist. Read your insurance policy carefully, and ask any professionals you plan to consult whether their services are covered by the terms of your policy.

4. Psychiatrists are M.D.'s who have received specialized training in the area of mental health. Many psychiatrists are interested in and trained to treat behavioral disorders and to use a variety of "talk therapies" in helping individuals function better. However, in general, most psychiatrists are especially trained in the use of medications for treating many forms of emotional and psychological difficulty, such as clinical depression.

5. Clinical social workers (M.S.W.'s) are trained to counsel in much the same way master's-level psychologists do. Some clinical social workers receive advanced training in counseling and earn certification by the Academy of Certified Social Workers (ACSW).

6. Pastoral counselors are ministers who have received advanced training in pastoral counseling. Such professionals are trained in various aspects of mental health and can specialize in individual, family, or group psychotherapy. Many pastoral counselors also have degrees in either social work or psychology.

7. It might be useful to consult a therapist who has a communicative relationship with your primary care physician. This

will ensure coordination of your physical and emotional care. Ask your doctor for advice and referral.

8. Above all else, trust your own instincts and impressions in deciding whether to continue with a particular therapist. No two therapists counsel in exactly the same way. What you get from different therapists will differ according to the "goodness of fit" between your personality and that of the therapist. If you do not like your therapist, find another one. *Your* health and happiness are at stake, not the feelings of the therapist.

Special guidelines are necessary for finding professional help to enhance your marriage.

1. Most mental health professionals receive very little training in marital and family therapy. Even fewer receive specific training in helping couples and families cope with physical illness. It is wise and appropriate to inquire about a given therapist's qualifications and experiences as a means of evaluating whether to hire him or her as your therapist. Ask the therapist the following questions:

   • Have you had specific training in marriage and family therapy?

   • Have you had experience in treating individuals and couples who are coping with heart illness or with other forms of chronic physical illness?

   • Are you treating such couples now?

   • What percentage of your practice is devoted to treating such couples?

   • What is your general theoretical orientation in conducting therapy?

   • Are you a certified marital and family therapist? (See below for details about certification.)

2. If an individual is defensive about answering the foregoing questions, find another therapist.

3. Choose a therapist whose orientation is primarily geared toward helping you to help each other solve your problems.

Psychoanalysis is interesting, but it is not particularly necessary in aiding you to cope better with heart illness as a couple or as individuals.

4. No universally accepted form of certification for marital and
family therapists exists, but a safe bet is to find a therapist
who either has Clinical Member or Supervisor status in the
American Association of Marriage and Family Therapy
(AAMFT). For a list of such therapists in your area, write or
call

AAMFT
1100 17th Street, NW
Washington, DC 20036-4601
(202) 452-0109

5. Marital support group programs are also available in many
communities. These programs typically consist of four- to
six-couple support groups who meet monthly to facilitate
each couple's attempts to remain lovingly connected. The
best-known such program is the Association of Couples for
Marital Enrichment (ACME). For a list of ACME contact persons in your area, write or call

ACME
P.O. Box 10596
Winston-Salem, NC 27108
(919) 724-1526

6. Many churches offer weekend marital enrichment programs
that can be very helpful in improving marital communications. Check with your local Mental Health Association for
descriptions of these and other options that may be available.

Recommended Reading

. . . . . .

Improving Marriage and Family Life

Beck, A. *Love Is Never Enough.* New York: Harper & Row, 1988.

Helmering, D. *Happily Ever After.* New York: Warner Books, 1986.

Hendrix, H. *Getting the Love You Want: A Guide for Couples.* New York: Harper & Row, 1988.

Lerner, H. *The Dance of Anger: A Woman's Guide to Changing the Patterns of Intimate Relationships.* New York: Harper & Row, 1985.

Mace, D., and Mace, V. *How to Have a Happy Marriage.* Nashville, Tenn.: Abingdon, 1977.

Paul, J., and Paul, M. *Do I Have to Give Up Me to Be Loved by You?* Minneapolis: CompCare, 1983.

Scarf, M. *Intimate Partners: Patterns in Love and Marriage.* New York: Random House, 1987.

Stuart, R., and Jacobson, B. *Second Marriage.* New York: W. W. Norton, 1985.

Sexual Aspects of Marriage

Barbach, L. *For Each Other.* New York: Signet, 1984.

Gochros, H., and Fisher, J. *Treat Yourself to a Better Sex Life.* Englewood Cliffs, N.J.: Spectrum, 1986.

Heiman, J.; LoPiccolo, L.; and LoPiccolo, J. *Becoming Orgasmic: A Sexual Growth Program for Women.* New York: Prentice-Hall, 1976.

Rosenthal, S. *Sex over Forty.* Los Angeles: Jeremy P. Tarcher, 1987.

Zilbergeld, B. *Male Sexuality.* New York: Bantam Books, 1978.

Type A Behavior Pattern

Friedman, M., and Rosenman, R. *Type A Behavior and Your Heart.* New York: Alfred A. Knopf, 1974.

Friedman, M., and Ulmer, D. *Treating Type A Behavior and Your Heart.* New York: Alfred A. Knopf, 1984.

Williams, R. *The Trusting Heart: Great News about Type A Behavior.* New York: Time Books, 1989.

Stress Management

Benson, H. *The Relaxation Response.* New York: William Morrow, 1975.

Maddi, S., and Kobasa, S. *The Hardy Executive: Health under Stress.* Homewood, Ill.: Dow Jones-Irwin, 1984.

Roskies, E. *Stress Management for the Healthy Type A: Theory and Practice.* New York: Guilford Press, 1987.

Attitudes, Emotions, and Health

Benson, H. *The Mind/Body Effect: How Behavioral Medicine Can Show You the Way to Better Health.* New York: Simon & Schuster, 1979.

Cousins, N. *Head First: The Biology of Hope.* New York: Dutton, 1989.

Siegel, B. *Peace, Love, and Healing—Bodymind Communication and the Path to Self-Healing: An Exploration.* New York: Harper & Row, 1990.

Simonton, W.; Matthews-Simonton, S.; and Creighton, J. *Getting Well Again.* Los Angeles: Jeremy P. Tarcher, 1978.

Cardiac Rehabilitation

Farquhar, J. *The American Way of Life Need Not Be Hazardous to Your Health: Coping with Life's Seven Major Risk Factors.* Reading, Mass.: Addison-Wesley Publishing Co., 1987.

Kwiterovich, P. *Beyond Cholesterol: The Johns Hopkins Complete Guide for Avoiding Heart Disease.* Baltimore: Johns Hopkins University Press, 1989.

Nutrition

Brody, J. *Jane Brody's Nutrition Book.* New York: Bantam Books, 1982.

DeBakey, M.; Gotto, A. M.; Scott, L. W.; and Foreyt, J. P. *The Living Heart Diet.* New York: Simon & Schuster, 1986.

Nash, J. *Taking Charge of Your Weight and Well-being.* 2nd ed. Menlo Park, Calif.: Bull Pub., 1989.

Personal Narratives about Heart Disease

Budnick, H. *Heart to Heart: Understanding the Emotional Aspects of Heart Disease.* Santa Fe, N.Mex.: Health Press, 1990.

Castelli, J. *I'm Too Young to Have a Heart Attack.* Rocklin, Calif.: Prima Publishing and Communications, 1990.

Cousins, N. *The Healing Heart: Antidotes to Panic & Helplessness.* Guilford, Conn.: Norton, 1983.

King, L., and Colen, B. *Mr. King, You're Having a Heart Attack: How a Heart Attack and Bypass Surgery Changed My Life.* New York: Delacorte, 1989.

Levin, R. *Heartmates: A Survival Guide for the Cardiac Spouse.* New York: Pocket Books, 1987.

Family Issues in Coping with Chronic Illness

Kievman, B. *For Better or for Worse: A Couple's Guide to Dealing with Chronic Illness.* Chicago: Contemporary Books, 1989.

Simonton, S. *The Healing Family: The Simonton Approach for Families Facing Illness.* New York: Bantam Books, 1984.

Strong, M. *Mainstay: For the Well Spouse of the Chronically Ill.* New York: Penguin, 1988.

References

■ ■ ■ ■ ■

Adsett, C., and Bruhn, J. Short-term group psychotherapy for post-myocardial infarction patients and their wives. *Canadian Medical Association Journal* 99, no. 12 (1968): 577–84.

Alberti, R., and Emmons, M. *A Guide to Assertive Living: Your Perfect Right.* San Luis Obispo, Calif.: Impact Publishers, 1982.

Anderson, B., and Wolf, F. Chronic physical illness and sexual behaviors: psychological issues. *J. of Consulting and Clinical Psychology* 54, no. 2 (1986): 168–75.

Andrew, G.; Oldridge, N.; Parker, J.; Cunningham, D.; Rechnitzer, P.; Jones, N.; Buck, C.; Kavanagh, T.; Shepherd, R.; Sutton, J.; and McDonald, W. Reasons for dropout from exercise programs in post coronary patients. *Med. Sci. Sports Exerc.* 11 (1979): 376–78.

Baggs, J., and Karch, A. Sexual counseling of women with coronary heart disease. *Heart Lung* 16 (1987): 154–59.

Bar-On, D., and Cristal, M. D. Causal attributions of patients, their spouses and physicians, and the rehabilitation of the patients after their first myocardial infarction. *J. Cardiopulmonary Rehabil.* 7 (1987): 285–98.

Beach, S. R., and O'Leary, K. D. The treatment of depression occurring in the context of marital discord. *Behavior Therapy* 17 (1986): 43–49.

Ben-Sira, Z., and Eliezer, R. The structure of readjustment after heart attack, *Soc. Sci. Med.* 30, no. 5 (1990): 523–36.

Berkman, L., and Seeman, T. The influence of social relationships on aging and the development of cardiovascular disease: A review. *Postgrad. Med. J.* 62: (August 1986), 805–7.

Berkman, L., and Syme, S. Social networks, host resistance and mortality: A nine-year follow-up of Alameda County residents. *Am. J. Epidemiol.* 109 (1979): 186–204.

Blackford, K. The children of chronically ill parents. *J. of Psychosocial Nursing & Mental Health Services* 26, no. 3 (1988): 33–36.

Blaney, N. T.; Brown, P.; and Blaney, P. H. Type A, marital adjustment, and life stress. *J. of Behavioral Medicine* 9, no. 5 (1986): 491–502.

Bloch, A., and Maeder, J. Sexual problems of myocardial infarction. *Am. Heart J.* 90 (1975): 536–37.

Blumenthal, J.; Emery, C. F.; and Rejeski, W. J. The effects of exercise and psychosocial functioning after myocardial infarction. *J. Cardiopulmonary Rehabil.* 8 (1988): 183–93.

Boone, T., and Kelley, R. Sexual issues and research in counseling the postmyocardial infarction patient. *J. Cardiovasc. Nurs.* 4, no. 4 (1990): 65–75.

Bouras, N.; Vanger, P.; and Bridges, P. Marital problems in chronically depressed and physically ill patients and their spouses. *Comprehensive Psychiatry* 27, no. 2 (1986): 127–30.

Bowen, M. *The Family in Clinical Practice.* Northvale, N.J.: Jason Aronson, 1978.

Brackney, B. The impact of home hemodialysis on the marital dyad. *J. of Mar. and Fam. Ther.* 5, no. 1 (1979): 55–60.

Bradley, W. New techniques in evaluation of impotence. *Urology* 39 (1987): 383–88.

Bray, G.; DeFrank, R.; and Wolfe, T. Sexual functioning in stroke survivors. *Arch. Phys. Med. Rehabil.* 62 (1981): 286–88.

Brenton, M. *Sex and Your Heart.* New York: Coward-McCann, 1968.

Brownell, K.; Heckerman, C.; Westlake, R.; Hayes, S.; and Monti, P. The effect of couples training and partner cooperativeness in behavioral treatment of obesity. *Behav. Res. Ther.* 16 (1978): 323–33.

Burgess, A., and Hartman, C. Patients' perceptions: Key to recovery. *Am. J. Nurs.* 86, no. 5 (1986): 568–71.

Burke, R.; Weir, T.; and DuWors, R. Type A behavior of administrators and wives' reports of marital satisfaction and well-being. *J. of Applied Psychology* 64, no. 1 (1979): 57–65.

Burling, T. A.; Singleton, E. G.; Bigelow, G. E.; Baile, W. F.; and Gottlieb, S. H. Smoking following myocardial infarction: A critical review of the literature. *Health Psychology* 3, no. 1 (1984): 83–96.

Burnett, W., and Chahine, R. Sexual dysfunction as a complication of propranolol therapy in men. *Cardiovascular Medicine* 4 (1979): 811–15.

Burns, D. *Feeling Good: The New Mood Therapy.* New York: New American Library, 1980.

Bursten, B. Family dynamics, the sick role, and medical hospital admission. *Family Process* 4 (1965): 206–16.

Campbell, S. *Beyond the Power Struggle: Dealing with Conflict in Love and Work.* San Luis Obispo, Calif.: Impact Publishers, 1984.

_____. *The Couple's Journey: Intimacy as a Path to Wholeness.* San Luis Obispo, Calif.: Impact Publishers, 1982.

Caplan, J.; Manuck, S.; Clarkson, T.; Lusso, F.; Taub, D.; and Miller, E. Social stress and atherosclerosis in normocholesterolemic monkeys. *Sciences* 220 (1983): 733.

Carmelli, D.; Swan, G. E.; and Rosenman, R. H. The relationship between wives' social and psychologic status and their husbands' coronary heart disease. *Amer. J. of Epidemiology* 122, no. 1 (1985): 90–100.

Carmignani, G.; Corbu, C.; Pirozzi, F.; DeStefani, S.; and Spano, G. Cavernous artery revascularization in vasculogenic impotence: New simplified technique. *Urology* 30 (1987): 23–26.

Carpenter, J. Changing roles and disagreements in families with disabled husbands. *Archives of Physical Medical Rehabilitation* 55 (1974): 272–74.

Cassileth, B.; Lusk, E.; Miller, D.; Brown, L.; and Miller, C. Psychosocial correlates of survival in advanced malignant disease. *New England Journal of Medicine* 312, no. 24 (1985): 1551–70.

Chandra, V.; Szklo, M.; Goldberg, R.; and Tonascia, J. The impact of marital status on survival after acute myocardial infarction: A population based study. *Amer. J. of Epidem.* 117 (1983): 320.

Chapple, E. *Culture and Biological Man,* New York: Holt, Rinehart, and Winston, 1970.

Cleveland, M. *Living Well: A Twelve-Step Response to Chronic Illness and Disability.* New York: Harper & Row, 1988.

Cohen, F. Personality, stress, and the development of physical illness. In *Health Psychology: A Handbook,* edited by G. Stone; F. Cohen; and N. Adler. San Francisco: Jossey-Bass, 1980.

_____, and Lazarus, R. Coping with the stresses of illness. In *Health Psychology: A Handbook,* edited by G. Stone; F. Cohen; and N. Adler. San Francisco: Jossey-Bass, 1980.

Cohen, S., and Syme, S., eds. *Social Support and Health.* New York: Academic Press, 1985.

Comfort, A. *Sexual Consequences of Disability.* Philadelphia: George F. Stickly, 1978.

Coppotelli, H. C., and Orleans, C. T. Partner support and other determinants of smoking cessation maintenance among women. *J. of Consulting and Clinical Psychology* 53, no. 4 (1985): 455–60.

Crawshaw, J. Community rehabilitation after acute myocardial infarction. *Heart and Lung* 3 (1974): 258.

Croog, S., and Fitzgerald, E. Subjective stress and serious illness of a spouse: Wives of heart patients. *J. of Health and Soc. Behav.* 19, no. 2 (1978): 166–78.

Croog, S., and Levine, S. *The Heart Patient Recovers: Social and Psychological Factors.* New York: Human Sciences Press, 1977.

_____, and Levine, S. *Life After a Heart Attack: Social and Psychological Factors 8 Years Later.* New York: Human Sciences Press, 1982.

D'Afflitti, J., and Weitz, W. Rehabilitating the stroke patient through patient-family groups. *Int. J. of Group Psychotherapy* 25, no. 3 (1974): 323–32.

Daltroy, L., and Godin, G. Spouse intention to encourage cardiac patient participation in exercise. *Amer. J. of Health Promotion* 4, no. 1 (1989): 12–17.

Davidson, D. M. Social support and cardiac rehabilitation: A review. *J. of Cardiopulmonary Rehabil.* 7 (1987): 196–200.

Delvey, J., and Hopkins, L. Pain patients and their partners: The role of collusion in chronic pain. *J. Mar. and Fam. Ther.* 8, no. 1 (1982): 135–42.

Derogatis, L., and King, K. The coital coronary: A reassessment of the concept. *Arch. Sex. Behav.* 10 (1981): 325–35.

Dhooper, S. Social networks and support during the crisis of heart attack. *Health Soc. Work* 9 (1984): 294–303.

Doehrman, S. Psychosocial aspects of recovery from coronary heart disease: A review. *Soc. Sci. Med.* 11 (1977): 199–218.

Dracup, K.; Meleis, A.; Baker, K.; and Ilefsen, P. E. Family focused cardiac rehabilitation: A role supplementation program for cardiac patients and spouses. *Nur. Clin. of N. Amer.* 19 (1984): 113–23.

Dunlap, W., and Hollinsworth, J. How does a handicapped child affect the family? Implications for practitioners. *The Family Coordinator* 26, no. 2 (1977): 286–93.

Eaker, E.; Haynes, S.; and Feinleib, M. Spouse behavior and coronary heart disease: Prospective results from the Framingham Heart Study. *Activities Nervosa Superior* 25, no. 2 (1983): 81–90.

———. Spouse behavior and coronary heart disease in men: Prospective results from the Framingham heart study. II. Modification of risk in Type A husbands according to the social and psychological status of their wives. *Amer. J. of Epidemiology* 118, no. 1 (1983): 23–41.

Earp, J. A.; Ory, M. G.; and Strogatz, D. S. The effects of family involvement and practitioner home visits on the control of hypertension. *Amer. J. of Public Health* 72, no. 10 (1982): 1146–54.

Eckberg, J.; Griffith, N.; and Foxall, M. Spouse burnout syndrome. *J. of Advanced Nur.* 11, no. 2 (1986): 161–65.

Eliot, R. What families can do to help CV recovery. *Behavioral Medicine* 6 (1979): 21–23.

Ellis, A., and Harper, R. *A New Guide to Rational Living.* North Hollywood: Wilshire Book Co., 1975.

Emery, C. F.; Pinder, S. L.; and Blumenthal, J. A. Psychological effects of exercise among elderly cardiac patients. *J. of Cardiopulmonary Rehabil.* 9 (1989): 46–53.

Engel, G.; Burnham, S.; and Carter, M. Penile blood pressure in the evaluation of erectile impotence. *Fertility and Sterility* 30 (1978): 687–90.

Evans, P. Type A behavior and coronary heart disease: When will the jury return? *Brit. J. of Psychology* 81, no. 2 (1990): 147–57.

Fink, S.; Skipper, J.; and Hallenbeck, P. Physical disability and problems in marriage. *J. of Mar. and the Fam.* 30 (1968): 64–73.

Fisher, H. Management of emotional factors in coronary disease. *Psychosomatics* 18, no. 4 (1977): 10–13.

Fox, M. *Original Blessing*. Santa Fe, N.Mex.: Bear & Co., 1983.

Foxall, M., and Ekberg, J. Loneliness of chronically ill adults and their spouses. *Issues in Mental Health Nursing* 10, no. 2 (1989): 149–67.

Foxall, M.; Eckberg, J.; and Griffith, N. Spousal adjustment to chronic illness. *Rehabilitation Nursing* 11, no. 2 (1986): 13–16.

Frankl, V. *Man's Search for Meaning*. New York: Touchstone, 1984.

Friedman, J. Sexual adjustment of the postcoronary male. In *Handbook of Sex Therapy*, edited by J. LoPiccolo and L. LoPiccolo. New York: Plenum, 1978.

Friedman, M.; Thoresen, C. E.; Gill, J. J.; Powell, L. H.; Ulmer, D.; Thompson, L.; Price, V. A.; Rabin, D. D.; Breall, W. S.; Dixon, T.; Levy, R.; and Bourg, E. Alteration of Type A behavior and reduction in cardiac recurrences in postmyocardial infarction patients. *American Heart Journal* 108, no. 2 (1984): 237–48.

Friis, R., and Armstrong, G. Social support and social networks, and coronary heart disease and rehabilitation. *J. of Cardiopulmonary Rehabil.* 6 (1986): 132–47.

Fuentes, P.; Rosenberg, J.; and Marks, R. Sexual side effects: What to tell your patients, what not to say. *RN* 46, no. 2 (February 1983): 35–41.

Gentry, D., and Williams, R. eds. *Psychological Aspects of a Myocardial Infarction and Coronary Care*, St. Louis: C. V. Mosby, 1975.

Gentry, W.; Baider, L.; Deter Oude-Weme, J.; Musch, F.; and Gary, H. Type A/B differences in coping with acute myocardial infarction: Further consideration. *Heart Lung* 12 (1983): 212–19.

Gentry, W.; Aronson, M.; Blumenthal, J.; Costa, P.; and DiGiacomo, J. Cardiovascular disease in the elderly: Behavioral, cognitive and emotional considerations. *J. of the Amer. Coll. of Cardiology* 10, no. 2, suppl. A (1987): 38A–41A.

Giacquinta, B. Helping families face the crisis of cancer. *Amer. J. of Nursing* 77, no. 10 (1977): 1585–88.

Giese, H., and Schomer, H. H. Life-style changes and mood profile of cardiac patients after an exercise rehabilitation program. *J. Cardiopulmonary Rehabil.* 6 (1986): 30–37.

Gilbert, D.; Hagen, R.; and D'Agostino, J. The effects of cigarette smoking on human sexual potency. *Addictive Behaviors* 11 (1986): 431–34.

Goldberg, S.; Morris, P.; Simans, R.; Fowler, S.; Levison, H. Chronic illness in infancy and parenting stress: A comparison of three groups of parents. *J. of Pediatric Psych.* 15, no. 3 (1990): 347–58.

Goodwin, J.; Hunt, W.; Key, C.; and Samet, J. The effect of marital status on stage, treatment and survival of cancer patients. *JAMA* 258, no. 21 (1987) 3125–3130.

Goulding, M., and Goulding, R. *Not to Worry: How to Free Yourself from Unnecessary Anxiety and Channel Your Worries into Positive Action*. New York: William Morrow, 1989.

Green, A. Sexual activity and the postmyocardial infarction patient. *Am. Heart J.* 89 (1975): 246–54.

Griffith, J., and Griffith, M. Structural family therapy in chronic illness: Intervention can help produce a more adaptive family structure. *Psychosomatics* 28, no. 4 (1987): 202–205.

Grinder, J., and Bandler, R. *France-Formations: Neuro-Linguistic Programming and the Structure of Hypnosis.* Moab, Utah: Real People Press, 1981.

Grolnick, L. A family perspective of psychosomatic factors in illness: A review of the literature. *Fam. Process* 11 (1972): 457–86.

Hackett, T. P. Depression following myocardial infarction. *Psychosomatics* 26, no. 11 (1985): 23–28.

Haley, J., and Hoffman, L. *Techniques of Family Therapy.* New York: Basic Books, 1967.

Halperin, J., and Levine, R. *Bypass.* New York: Random House, 1985.

Haywood, J., and Obier, K. Psycho-social problems of coronary care unit patients. *J. Nat. Med. Assoc.* 63 (1971): 425–28.

Heinzelmann, F., and Bagley, R. Response to physical activity programs and their effect on health behaviors. *Public Health Rep.* 85 (1970): 905–11.

Hellerstein, H., and Friedman, E. Sexual activity and the post-coronary patient. *Arch. Intern. Med.* 125 (1970): 187–99.

Henley, A., and Williams, R. Type A and B subjects' self-reported cognitive/affective/behavioral responses to descriptions of potentially frustrating situations. *J. Hum. Stress* 12 (1986): 168–74.

Hilbert, G. Spouse support and myocardial infarction patient compliance. *Nursing Research* 34, no. 4 (1985): 217–20.

Hoffman, L. *Foundations of Family Therapy: A Conceptual Framework for Systems Change.* New York: Basic Books, 1981.

Hoffman, N. *Change of Heart: The Bypass Experience.* New York: Harcourt Brace Jovanovich, 1985.

Holahan, C. J., and Moos, R. H. Life stress and health: Personality, coping, and family support in stress resistance. *J. of Person. and Soc. Psych.* 49, no. 3 (1985): 739–47.

———. Personality, coping, and family resources in stress resistance: A longitudinal analysis. *J. of Person. and Soc. Psych.* 51, no. 2 (1986): 389–95.

Holmes, T. S., and Rahe, R. H. The social adjustment rating scale. *Psychosomatic Research* 11 (1967): 213–18.

Hooyman, N., and Lustbader, W. *Taking Care: Supporting Older People and Their Families.* New York: The Free Press, 1986.

Hudgens, A. Family-oriented treatment of chronic pain. *J. of Mar. and Fam. Ther.* 5, no. 4 (1979): 67–78.

Jenkins, C. D. Psychologic and social precursors of coronary disease. *New England Journal of Medicine* 284 (1971): 244–55.

Johnston, B.; Cantwell, J.; Watt, E.; and Fletcher, G. Sexual activity in exercising patients after myocardial infarction and revascularization. *Heart Lung* 7 (1978): 1026–31.

Johnson, S. *The Precious Present*. New York: Doubleday, 1981.

Kahler, T., and Capers, H. The miniscript. *Transactional Analysis Journal* 4, no. 1 (1974): 26–42.

Kaplan, D.; Smith, A.; Grobstein, R.; and Fischman, S. Family mediation of stress. *Social Work* 18 (July 1973): 60–69.

Katzin, L. Chronic illness and sexuality. *Amer. J. of Nursing* 90, no. 1 (1990): 54–59.

Kerr, M., and Bowen, M. *Family Evaluation: An Approach Based on Bowen Theory*. New York: W. W. Norton & Co., 1988.

Kiecolt-Glaser, J.; Fisher, L.; Ogrocki, P.; Stout, J.; Speicher, C.; and Glaser, R. Marital quality, marital disruption, and immune function. *Psychosomatic Medicine*, 49 (1987): 13–33.

Kiecolt-Glaser, J.; Williger, D.; Stout, J.; Messick, G.; Sheppard, S.; Richer, D.; Romisher, S.; Briner, W.; Bonnell, G.; and Donnerberg, R. Psychosocial enhancement of immunocompetence in a geriatric population. *Health Psychology* 4 (1985): 25–41.

Kinsey, M. G.; Fletcher, B. J.; Rice, C. R.; Watson, P.H.; and Fletcher, G. F. Coronary risk factor modification followed by home-monitored exercise in coronary bypass surgery patients: A four-year follow-up study. *J. Cardiopulmonary Rehabil.* 9 (1989): 207–12.

Kline, N., and Warren, B. The relationship between husband and wife perceptions of the prescribed health regimen and level of function in the marital couple post-myocardial infarction. *Family Practice Research Journal* 2, no. 4 (1983): 271–80.

Klinger, M. Compliance and the post-MI patient. *Can. Nurs.* 80, no. 7 (1984): 32–37.

Knafl, K., and Deatrick, J. How families manage chronic conditions: An analysis of the concept of normalization. *Research in Nursing & Health* 9(3): 215–22 (September 1986).

Kolman, P. Sexual dysfunction in the post-MI patient. *J. of Cardiac Rehabilitation* 4 (1984): 334–40.

Kolodny, R.; Masters, W.; and Johnson, V. *Textbook of Sexual Medicine*. Boston: Little, Brown, 1979.

Krantz, D. Cognitive processes and recovery from heart attack: A review and theoretical analysis. *J. Hum. Stress* 6 (1980): 27–38.

————, ed. Stress management: An important behavioral medicine contribution to cardiac rehabilitation. *J. Cardiopulm. Rehab.* 5 (1985): 207–267.

Krantz, D. S., and Durel, L. A. Psychobiological substrates of the Type A behavior pattern. *Health Psychology* 2, no. 4 (1983): 393–411.

Kreeft, P. *Making Sense out of Suffering*. New York: Walker and Co., 1986.

Kulik, J., and Mahler, H. Social support and recovery from surgery. *Health Psychology* 8, no. 2 (1989): 221–38.

Kushner, H. *When Bad Things Happen to Good People*. New York: Avon Books, 1981.

Lambert, C., and Lambert, V. Psychosocial impacts created by chronic illness. *Nur. Clin. of N. Amer.* 22, no. 3 (1987): 527–33.

Lancaster, L. Impact of chronic illness over the life span. *Ana Journal* 15, no. 3 (1988): 164–68.

Langeluddecke, P.; Tennant, C.; Fulcher, G.; Barid, D.; Hughes, C. Coronary artery bypass surgery: Impact upon the patient's spouse. *J. of Psychosomatic Research* 33, no. 2 (1989): 155–59.

Larkin, J. Factors influencing one's ability to adapt to chronic illness. *Nur. Clin. of N. Amer.* 22, no. 3 (1987): 535–42.

Lazarus, A. *Multimodal Behavior Therapy.* New York: Springer, 1976.

Levenson, F. *The Anti-Cancer Marriage: Living Longer Through Loving.* New York: Stein and Day, 1982.

Levy, S. Emotions and the progression of cancer: A review. *Advances: J. of the Institute for the Advancement of Health* 1, no. 1 (1984): 10–15.

Levy, S.; Lee, J.; Bagley, C.; and Lippman, M. Survival hazards analysis in recurrent breast cancer patients: Seven-year follow-up *Psychosomatic Medicine* 50 (1988): 520–28.

Locke, S., and Colligan, D. *The Healer Within: The New Medicine of Mind and Body.* New York: New American Library, 1987.

Lynch, J. *The Language of the Heart: The Body's Response to Human Dialogue.* New York: Basic Books, 1985.

Madanes, C., and Haley, J. Dimensions of family therapy. *J. of Nervous and Mental Disease* 165, no. 1 (1977): 88–98.

Massie, E.; Rose, E.; and Rupp, S. Viewpoints: Sudden death during coitus— fact or fiction? *Medical Aspects of Human Sexuality* 3 (1969): 22–26.

Mathews, K. A. Psychological perspectives on the Type A behavior pattern. *Psychological Bulletin* 91, no. 2 (1982): 292–323.

Maurer, J., and Strasberg, P. *Building a New Dream: A Family Guide to Coping with Chronic Illness & Disability.* Reading, Mass.: Addison-Wesley, 1989.

Mayou, R. The course and determinants of myocardial infarction. *Brit. J. of Psychia.* 134 (June 1979): 588–94.

———. Effectiveness of cardiac rehabilitation. *J. Psychosom. Res.* 25, no. 5 (1981): 423–27.

———. Prediction of emotional and social outcome after a heart attack. *J. Psychosom. Res.* 28 (1984): 17–25.

———; Foster, A.; and Williamson, B. Psychosocial adjustment in patients one year after myocardial infarction. *J. Psychosom. Res.* 22 (1978): 447–53.

McClelland, D. Some reflections on the two psychologies of love. *J. of Personality* 54 (1986): 2–10.

McCubbin, H.; Joy, C.; Cauble, A.; Comeau, J.; Patterson, J.; and Needle, R. Family stress and coping: A decade review. *J. Mar. and the Family* 42, no. 4 (1980): 855–71.

———, and Figley, C. *Stress and the Family: Coping With Normative Transitions.* New York: Brunner/Mazel, 1983.

_____. *Stress and the Family: Coping With Catastrophe*. New York: Brunner/Mazel, 1983.

Medalie, J.; Snyder, M.; and Groen, J. Angina pectoris among 10,000 men: 5-year incidence and univariate analysis. *Am. J. Med.* 55 (1973): 583–87.

Mercer, R. Response to "Life-span development: A review of theory and practice for families with chronically ill members." *Scholarly Inquiry For Nursing Practice* 3, no. 1 (1989): 23–27.

Meyer, K., and Weidemann, H. Coronary risk factors and their relations to somatic and psychosocial factors in female patients with myocardial infarction. *J. Cardiopulmonary Rehabil.* 9 (1989): 164–172.

Miller, J., and Janosik, E. *Family-Focused Care*. New York: McGraw-Hill, 1980.

Miller, N. H.; Taylor, C. B.; Davidson, D. M.; Hill, M. N.; and Krantz, D. S. The efficacy of risk factor intervention and psychosocial aspects of cardiac rehabilitation. *J. of Cardiopulmonary Rehabil.* 10 (1990): 198–209.

Miller, R., and Lefcourt, H. Social intimacy: An important moderator of stressful life events. *Am. J. Commun. Psychol.* 11 (1983): 127–39.

Minuchin, S. *Families and Family Therapy*. Cambridge, Mass.: Harvard Univ. Press, 1974.

_____; Haker, L.; Rosman, B.; Liebman, R.; Milman, L.; and Todd, T. A conceptual model for psychosomatic illness in children: Family organization and family therapy. *Archives of General Psychiatry* 32 (1975): 1031–36.

_____; Rosman, B.; and Baker, L. *Psychosomatic Families: Anorexia Nervosa in Context*. Cambridge, Mass.: Harvard Univ. Press, 1978.

Moos, R., and Tsy, U. The crisis of physical illness: An overview. In *Coping With Physical Illness*, edited by R. Moos. New York: Plenum Medical Book Co., 1977.

Murray, G., and Beller, G. Cardiac rehabilitation following coronary artery bypass surgery. *Am. Heart J.* 105 (1983): 1009–18.

O'Farrell, T. J.; Cutter, H. S. G.; and Floyd, F. J. Evaluating behavioral marital therapy for male alcoholics: Effects on marital adjustment and communication from before to after treatment. *Behavior Therapy* 16 (1985): 147–67.

Oldridge, N. B. Compliance and dropout in cardiac exercise rehabilitation. *J. of Cardiac Rehabil.* 4 (1984): 166–77.

Ornish, D. *Dr. Dean Ornish's Program for Reversing Heart Disease*. New York: Random House, 1990.

Packa, D.; Branyon, M.; Kinney, M.; Khan, S.; Kelley, R.; Miers, L. Quality of life of elderly patients enrolled in cardiac rehabilitation programs. *J. Cardiovasc. Nurs.* 3, no. 2 (1989): 33–42.

Papadopoulos, C. A survey of sexual activity after MI. *Cardiovascular Medicine* 3 (1978): 821–26.

Patterson, J. Illness beliefs as a factor in patient-spouse adaptation to treatment for coronary artery disease. *Family Systems Medicine* 7, no. 4 (1989): 428–42.

Pearce, J. W.; LeBow, M. D.; and Orchard, J. Role of spouse involvement in the behavioral treatment of overweight women. *J. of Consulting and Clinical Psychology* 49, no. 2 (1981): 236–44.

Peck. S. *The Road Less Traveled: A New Psychology of Love, Traditional Values and Spiritual Growth.* New York: Simon and Schuster, 1978.

Peterson, C.; Seligman, M.; and Vaillant, G. Pessimistic explanatory style is a risk factor for physical illness: A thirty-five-year longitudinal study. *J. of Personality and Social Psychol.* 55, no. 1 (1988): 23–27.

Peterson, Y. The impact of physical disability on marital adjustment: A literature review. *Family Coordinator* 28, no. 1 (1979): 47–51.

Powell, L. H.; Friedman, M.; Thoresen, C. E.; Gill, J. J.; and Ulmer, D. K. Can the Type A behavior pattern be altered after myocardial infarction? A second year report from the recurrent coronary prevention project. *Psychosomatic Medicine* 46, no. 4 (1984): 293–313.

Power, P. The adolescent's reaction to chronic illness of a parent: Some implications for family counseling. *Int. J. of Family Counseling* 5 (1977): 70–78.

Price, V. *Type A Behavior Pattern: A Model for Research and Practice.* San Diego, Calif.: Academic Press, 1982.

Rankin, S., and Weekes, D. Life-span development: A review of theory and practice for families with chronically ill members. *Scholarly Inquiry for Nursing Practice* 3, no. 1 (1989): 3–22.

Rauch, J., and Kneen, K. Accepting the gift of life: Heart transplants' postoperative adaptive tasks. *Soc. Wk. in Health Care* 14, no. 1 (1989): 47–59.

Razin, A. Psychosocial intervention in coronary artery disease: A review. *Psychosomatic Med.* 44 (1982): 363–86.

Rejeski, J. Rehabilitation and prevention of coronary heart disease: An overview of Type A behavior pattern. *Quest* 33, no. 2 (1982): 154–65.

———; Morley, D.; and Sotile, W. Cardiac rehabilitation: A conceptual framework for psychologic assessment. *J. of Cardiac Rehabilitation* 5, no. 4 (1985): 172–80.

Rogers, K. Nature of spousal supportive behaviors that influence heart transplant patient compliance. *J. Heart Transplant* 6 (1987): 90–95.

Rolland, J. Chronic illness and the life cycle: A conceptual framework. *Family Process* 26, no. 2 (1987): 203–21.

———. Anticipatory loss: A family systems developmental framework. *Family Process* 29, no. 3 (1990): 229–44.

Rosen, J., and Bibring, G. Psychological reactions of hospitalized male patients to heart attack: Age and social-class differences. *Psychosomatic Medicine* 28 (1969): 808–21.

Roy, R. Marital and family issues in patients with chronic pain. *Psychotherapy and Psychosomatics* 37, no. 1 (1982): 1–12.

Rubberman, W.; Weinblatt, E.; Goldberg, J.; and Chaudhary, B. Psychosocial influences on mortality after myocardial infarction. *New England Journal of Medicine* 312 (1984): 552.

Satir, V. *Conjoint Family Therapy.* Palo Alto, Calif.: Science and Behavior Books, 1964.

_____. *Peoplemaking*. Palo Alto, Calif.: Science and Behavior Books, 1972.

Schaffer, W., and Cobb, E. Recurrent VF and modes of death in survivors of out-of-hospital VF. *New England Journal of Medicine* 293 (1975): 259–64.

Scheingold, L., and Wagner, N. *Sound Sex and the Aging Heart*. New York: Human Sciences Press, 1974.

Schmidt, T.; Dembroski, T.; and Blumchen, G., eds. *Biological and Psychological Factors in Cardiovascular Disease*. New York: Springer, 1987.

Schneiderman, N.; Chesney, M.; and Krantz, D. Biobehavioral aspects of cardiovascular disease: Progress and prospects. *Health Psychology* 8, no. 6 (1989): 649–76.

Schomer, H., and Noakes, T. The psychological effects of exercise training on patients after a myocardial infarction: A pilot study. *South Afr. Med. J.* 64 (1983): 473–75.

Schuman, S.; Jabaily, G.; and Samuelson, D. Life events in a family with life threatening illness. *Psychosomatics* 18 (1977): 34–39.

Seligman, M., *Learned Optimism*. New York: Alfred A. Knopf, 1990.

Shambaugh, P., and Kanter, S. Spouses under stress: Group meetings with spouses of patients on hemodialysis. *Amer. J. of Psychiatry* 125 (1969): 928–36.

Siegel, B. *Love, Medicine and Miracles: Lessons Learned about Self-Healing from a Surgeon's Experience with Exceptional Patients*. New York: Harper & Row, 1986.

Siegfried, H., coordinator. *The Heart Book: A Program for Prevention of Heart Attack from Researchers at the Duke University Medical Center*. New York: Delair Publishing Co., 1981.

Silberfarb, P., and Greer, S. Psychological concomitants of cancer: Clinical aspects. *Amer. J. of Psychotherapy* 36, no. 4 (1982): 470–78.

Singer, L.; Drotar, D.; and Doershuk, C. Psychosocial management of chronic lung disorders. *Pediatrician* 15, no. 1–2 (1988): 29–36.

Sirles, A., and Selleck, C. Cardiac disease and the family: Impact, assessment, and implications. *J. Cardiovasc. Nurs.* 3, no. 2 (1989): 23–32.

Sotile, W. The penile prosthesis: A review. *J. of Sex and Marital Therapy* 5 (1979): 90–102.

Southam, C. Emotions, immunology, and cancer: How might the psyche influence neoplasia? *Annals of the New York Academy of Sciences* 164 (1969): 473–75.

Speers, M. A.; Kasl, S. V.; and Ostfeld, A. M. Marital correlates of blood pressure. *Amer. J. of Epidemiology* 129, no. 5 (1989): 956–72.

Stern, M., and Cleary, P. The National Exercise and Heart Disease Project: Long-term psychosocial outcome. *Arch. Intern. Med.* 142 (1982): 1093–97.

Stewart, I., and Joines, V. *TA Today: A New Introduction to Transactional Analysis*. Nottingham, England: Lifespace Publishing, 1987.

Storer, J. H.; Frate, D.A.; Johnson, S. A.; and Greenberg, A. M. When the cure seems worse than the disease: Helping families adapt to hypertension treatment. *Family Relations* 36 (1987): 311–15.

Strauss, A. *Chronic Illness and the Quality of Life.* St. Louis: Mosby, 1975.

Swan, G.; Carmelli, D.; and Rosenman, R. Spouse-pair similarity on the California Psychological Inventory with reference to husband's coronary heart disease. *Psychosom. Med.* 48, no. 3–4 (1986): 172–86.

Taylor, C.; Bandura, A.; Ewart, C.; Miller, N.; and Debusk, R. Exercise testing to enhance wives' confidence in their husbands' cardiac capability soon after clinically uncomplicated acute myocardial infarction. *Am. J. Cardiol.* 55 (1985): 635–38.

Teismann, M., and Rodgers, B. A comparison of a traditional and a marital approach to rehabilitation counseling. *J. of Mar. and Fam. Ther.* 8, no. 2 (1982): 91–93.

Thomas, C. Precursors of premature disease and death: The predictive potential of habits and family attitudes. *Annals of Internal Medicine* 87 (1976): 653–58.

―――――, and Duszynski, K. Closeness to parents and the family constellation in a prospective study of five disease states: Suicide, mental illness, malignant tumor, hypertension, and coronary heart disease. *Johns Hopkins Medical Journal* 134 (1970): 251–70.

Thoresen, C. E.; Friedman, M.; Powell, L. H.; Gill, J. J.; and Ulmer, D. Altering the Type A behavior pattern in postinfarction patients. *J. Cardiopulmonary Rehabil.* 5 (1985): 258–66.

Ueno, M. The so-called coition death. *Japanese Journal of Legal Medicine* 17 (1963): 333–40.

Uniken Venema-Van Uden, M.; Zoeteweij, M.; Erdman, R.; Van den Berg, G.; Smeets, J.; Weeda, H.; Vermeulen, A.; Van Meurs-van Woezik, N.; Ebink, C. Medical, social and psychological recovery after cardiac rehabilitation. *J. Psychosom. Research* 33, no. 5 (1989): 651–56.

Vaillant, G. Health consequences of adaptation to life. *Amer. J. of Med.* 67 (November 1979): 732–34.

Vyden, J. *How to Prevent Your Next Heart Attack.* Englewood Cliffs, N.J.: Prentice Hall, 1988.

Wadden, T. Predicting treatment response to relaxation therapy for essential hypertension. *J. of Nervous and Mental Disease* 171, no. 11 (1983): 683–89.

Waltz, M. Marital context and post-infarction quality of life: Is it social support or something more? *Soc. Sci. Med.* 22 (1986): 791–805.

―――――, and Badura, B. Subjective health, intimacy and perceived self-efficacy after a heart attack: Predicting life quality five years afterwards. *Soc. Ind. Res.* 20 (1988): 303–332.

―――――; Badura, B.; Pfaff, H.; and Schott, T. Marriage and the psychological consequences of a heart attack: A longitudinal study of adaptation to chronic illness after 3 years. *Soc. Sci. Med.* 27, no. 2 (1988): 149–58.

Waring, E. Marriages of patients with psychosomatic illness. *General Hospital Psychiatry* 5, no. 1 (1983): 49–53.

Watzlawick, P., and Coyne, J. Depression following stroke: Brief, problem-focused family treatment. *Family Process* 19, no. 1 (1980): 13–18.

Weakland, J. Family somatics: A neglected edge. *Family Process* 16, no. 3 (1977): 263–72.

Weiner, H. *Psychobiology and Human Disease.* New York: American Elsevier, 1977.

Whitaker, J. *Reversing Heart Disease.* New York: Warner Books, 1988.

Wiklund, I.; Sanne, H.; Vedin, A.; and Wilhelmsson, C. Psychosocial outcome one year after a first myocardial infarction. *J. Psychosom. Res.* 28 (1984): 309–21.

Wishnie, H.; Hackett, T.; and Cassem, N. Psychological hazards of convalescence following myocardial infarction. *JAMA* 215, no. 8 (1971): 1292–96.

Wright, L.; Bell, J.; and Rock, B. Smoking behavior and spouses: A case report. *Fam. Sys. Med.* 7, no. 2 (1989): 158–71.

————, and Leahey, M., eds. *Families and Chronic Illness.* Springhouse, Pa.: Springhouse Corporation, 1987.

Yelin, E. The myth of malingering: Why individuals withdraw from work in the presence of illness. *Milbank Quarterly* 64, no. 4 (1986): 622–49.

Young, R. The family-illness intermesh: Theoretical aspects and their application. *Soc. Sci. Med.* 17 (1983): 395–98.

Zahn, M. Incapacity, impotence, and invisible impairment: The effects upon interpersonal relations. *J. of Health and Social Behavior* 14 (1973): 115–23.

Index

∎ ∎ ∎ ∎ ∎

Adaptive thinking, 240–45
Adrenaline, 170, 171, 219
Aggressiveness, 197–98, 213
Aging, 95; and sexual functioning, 102, 109, 113, 114, 131; and sexual response, 104, 121, 122, 123–26, 129
AIDS epidemic, 114
Alberti, R., 213
Alcohol, 37, 205, 227
Alcoholism, 53
Aldactone, 118, 119
Aldomet, 119, 120
All-or-Nothing thinking, 240
Alpha blockers, 119
American Association for Cardiovascular and Pulmonary Rehabilitation, 235, 259
American Association of Marriage and Family Therapy, 266
American Heart Association, 235, 259
American Lung Association, 235, 259
Anger, 43, 161, 165, 215, 251
Angina, 36, 42, 116, 127
Angiotensin-converting enzyme (ACE) inhibitors, 119, 120–21
Angry state, 178, 181–82
Anxiety, 10, 55; and personality drivers, 144, 145; and sexual functioning, 122, 130, 134, 135
Apresoline, 119, 120
Arrhythmia, 120
Arterial plaque, 232–33
Arthritis, 126
Assertiveness, 213
Association of Couples for Marital Enrichment, 266
Atherosclerosis, 123

Bandler, Richard, 231–32
Behavior modification, 211
Beta blockers, 119
Blocadren, 119
Blood pressure: sexual response and, 115, 116, 118, 120, 126; stress reactions, 170, 171, 208–9, 219, 228
Blood pressure medication: emotional side effects, 227–28, 242; sexual side effects, 117, 118–21, 227
Brain, 117, 126, 142
Burns, David, 239

Calan, 119
Calcium channel blockers, 119, 120
Cancer, 125, 220, 233
Capoten, 119

Cardiac Couples, 235, 260
Cardiac functioning, 36, 126–27
Cardiac rehabilitation, xv, 10, 11; family
    reactions to, 12, 27, 28–29, 35–37,
    46, 59; family triangulation and, 62,
    63; formal programs, 234–35, 259;
    marital intimacy and, 78, 99, 163,
    239, 252; and marital tension, 10, 26,
    27, 29, 57; medical advice, 26,
    33–34; patient's attitudes and, 36–37,
    42, 54, 221–22, 223, 239, 245–46;
    personality types and, 155, 156, 157;
    and sex, 100, 101–2, 117, 129; as
    stressor, 47, 52, 77–78, 220, 238;
    Type A personality and, 160, 162–63,
    164, 215
Cardiovascular system, 115, 219
Cardizem, 119
Catapres, 119, 120
Children: parental heart illness and,
    44–46, 49–50, 58; Type A parents
    and, 185, 193; Type A personality de-
    velopment, 175–77
Children, adult, 17; family triangulation,
    61, 62, 63–64, 69, 70; parental heart
    illness and, 46, 59, 60–61, 224; pa-
    rental marital tension and, 67–70,
    72–73
Cholesterol levels, 232–33
Clitoris, 112
Cognitive distortion, 239–46
Cognitive impairment, 259–60
Cognitive rehearsal, 231–32
Coma, 107
Communication: family triangles,
    67–68; honesty in, 31–32, 47; mari-
    tal, 85, 87–88
Competitiveness, 162; control of, 173,
    213–14; denial of, 197–98; in mar-
    riage, 193; women and, 177
Congestive heart failure, 104
Corgard, 119, 120
Coronary artery bypass surgery, 36, 42;
    case studies, 3, 6, 19, 23, 55–56, 122,
    123
Coronary artery disease, 165
Counseling, 6, 46, 69, 134, 197; marital
    therapy, 78, 98, 99, 256, 265–66;
    therapists, 263–66

Dance of Anger (Lerner), 70
Death, 250; families and, 42–43; fear of,
    9, 44; fear and sex, 114, 127; social
    support and, 202
Depressed state, 178, 180–82
Depression: in cardiac rehabilitation, 10,
    26–27, 29; case studies, 4, 5, 15–16,
    55–56, 64, 65, 122; medication for,
    264; medication side effects, 120; per-
    sonality drives and, 155; reaction to
    illness, 40, 41, 238; in spouses of Type
    A personalities, 191, 192, 195, 197
Dermatological problems, 220
Diabetes, 206, 220
Diagnosis, 41–42
Diet: family patterns and, 14; heart pa-
    tients and, 37, 120, 232–33; spouses
    and, 31; in stress reduction, 227
Differentiation, 83, 84
Discounting, 241–42
Diuretics, 118, 119
Dyazide, 119
Dysfunctional relationships, 86
Dyspareunia, 112, 113

Ellis, Albert, 237
Emmons, M., 213
Emotional management, 226
Emotional reactions, 237, 246
Emotional reasoning, 243–44
Endorphins, 205
Enduron, 119
Environmental stress, 207–9, 228
Esidrex, 119
Estrogen, 124
Estrogen replacement therapy, 125
Exercise, 37; capacity testing, 36, 116;
    personality drivers and, 155, 157; and
    sexual exertion, 115–16, 120, 127–28;
    in stress reduction, 227; thinking pat-
    terns and, 240; Type A personality
    and, 173, 205–6
Extramarital affairs, 91, 190

Families: balancing of commitments,
    223–24, 225; cognitive distortion and
    adaptive thinking, 239–45; family
    structure, 16–20; family teams,
    12–14, 40, 248; healthy reactions to

illness, 21–30, 38, 39, 73; heart illness stresses, xv–xvi, 6, 7, 9; honesty in communication, 30–33; intimacy and rehabilitation, 163, 216, 220; and personality development, 79, 175–77; poor coping with illness, 40–47, 53–59, 60, 250; stress and exaggeration of roles, 47–52, 156; triangular relations, 61–73; Type A personalities and, 172, 181–82; vicious circles, 15–16
Feeling Good: The New Mood Therapy (Burns), 239
Fortune-telling, 242–43
Fox, Matthew, 226
Frankl, Viktor E., 246
Friedman, Meyer, 160, 164, 202, 203, 204, 208, 211, 212

Gastrointestinal disturbance, 220
Genitourinary problems, 220
Getting the Love You Want (Hendrix), 142
God, 38, 249–50, 251
Grieving, 24–25, 41, 43
Grinder, John, 231–32
Guide to Assertive Living (Alberti and Emmons), 213
Guilt, 34, 144, 195
Gynecological examination, 113

Harvard University, 247
Headaches, 3, 19, 220
Heart attacks, 36; children and, 44; denial of, 153; and exercise capacity, 116; and sexual functioning, 100, 115, 116, 127, 130, 134; Type A personality and, 215
—case studies: attitudes toward rehabilitation, 54, 221, 222, 238–39; family reactions, 6–7, 13, 64; patient reactions, 6, 51, 54, 58–59, 148; spouse reactions, 3–4, 50–51, 58, 146
Heart illness, xv–xvi, 9–10, 11, 248–49, 256; cognitive impairment, 259–60; effects on children, 60, 62, 72; and estrogen therapy, 125; healthy family coping, 22, 25, 28–30, 33, 36–38; personality-based reactions, 143, 152–53; psychological reactions to,

8–9, 220; relaxation training and, 230–31, 232–33; and sexual functioning, 100–101, 102, 114, 115, 129, 131, 136; social support and, 202, 234; stress reduction and, 219, 221, 226–35; thinking patterns and, 239–47; Type A personality and, 161, 165, 171–72, 183; unhealthy family coping, 48, 51–52, 53–54, 55, 56, 57
Heartmates: A Survival Guide for the Cardiac Spouse (Levin), 224
Heart patients: adult children of, 60, 62, 63; attitudes toward rehabilitation, 36–37; balancing of responsibilities, 223, 224, 225; cognitive distortion and adaptive thinking, 239–45; exercise capacity, 36, 116; family reactions and, 12, 23–24, 25, 26, 28–30, 35, 42–43; life changes and, 229; medication and, 118; personality drivers and, 152–53, 154; sexual fears, 100–102, 126–27, 130; sexual functioning, 102, 104, 115, 116, 118; spouses and, 77–78, 83, 182, 184, 225; stress reactions, 8–9, 40, 49; Type A personality, 162–63, 182, 184, 202–3
Heart rate: exercise and, 205; in sexual response, 115, 116; in stress reaction, 170, 171, 219
Hendrix, Harville, 142
Holmes, Oliver Wendell, 198
Holmes, Thomas, 229
Hormone therapy, 104, 125
Hospitalization, 22, 26
Hostility: controlling and reducing, 210, 211, 213–14, 215; and family members, 165, 174; in reaction to illness, 43; in Type A personality, 161, 162, 165, 177, 197–98
Hurry sickness, 160, 177, 198, 212–13
Hydro-Diuril, 119
Hygroton, 119
Hypertension, 104, 125
Hysterectomy, 104

Illness, stress-related, 220
Immune system, 219–20, 233

Impotence, 110, 118, 130
Inderol, 119, 120
Inflammatory joint disease, 220
Ismelin, 119, 120
Isoptin, 119

Jenkins, C. David, 164
Johnson, Spencer, 256, 257
Johnson, Virginia, 107

Kushner, Harold S., 249, 250

Labeling and mislabeling, 244
Lasix, 119
Lerner, Harriet Goldhor, 70
Levin, Rhoda, 224
Lopressor, 119, 120

Magnification and minimization, 243
Male Sexuality (Zilbergeld), 131
Man's Search for Meaning (Frankl), 246
Marital therapy, 78, 98, 99, 256, 265–66
Marriage, 7, 256, 257; balancing of
    commitments, 223–24, 225; cardiac
    rehabilitation and, xvi–xvii, 35, 57,
    77–78, 239; and family relationships,
    6, 17–18, 24, 25–26, 29, 49, 55,
    56–57; heart illness stress and, 221,
    224; intimacy in, 85–99, 197, 201,
    248; intimacy and cardiac rehabilita-
    tion, 10–11, 73, 78, 99, 100–101, 163,
    252; sex drives in, 102–3, 105–6, 122;
    stages of, 79–85; triangular relation-
    ships and, 62, 63, 65, 67, 68–69; Type
    A behavior and, 162, 163–64, 168–70,
    172, 174; Type A marriage patterns,
    174, 183–84, 186–201
Masters, William, 107
Maxzide, 119
Medical advice, 26, 33
Medical care, 43, 45
Medical insurance, 264
Medication, 37, 264; emotional side ef-
    fects, 227–28; sexual side effects, 102,
    114, 117–21; side effects, 9, 23
Melancholia, 24
Men: sexual problems, 107, 110–11, 118,
    120; sexual response cycle, 104, 107,

108, 109, 124; Type A personalities,
    161, 184, 188
Menopause, 124–25
Metabolic energy testing (MET), 116
Migraine headaches, 3
Mind reading, 242
Minipress, 119, 120
Muscular tension, 208, 228

Naqua, 119
National Stroke Association, 260
Nervous system, 170–71, 176, 205, 227
Nitroglycerin, 117, 127

Oretic, 119
Orgasm: aging and, 124, 129; energy ex-
    ertion, 116; medication and, 117, 120;
    men, 108, 110–11; sex drive and, 106,
    107; women, 108, 109, 110, 111–12
Ornish, Dean, 232–33
"Our Healing Philosophy," 250–52
Overgeneralization, 240–41

Parents, 122; in family structure, 12, 17;
    illness and children, 44–45, 46, 72;
    marital relationship and children,
    60–61, 62, 63, 67–68, 69; Type A
    personality, 175–76, 185
*Peace, Love, and Healing—Bodymind Com-
    munication and the Path to Self-Healing*
    (Siegel), 226
Pelvic angiography, 126
Penis, 109, 112, 124, 126
Perfectionism, 161, 162, 191
Personality, 141–42, 176; driver types,
    143–52; and heart illness reactions,
    143, 152–59; and sexual behavior,
    133–34
Personalization of blame, 245
Peterson, Christopher, 247
Physical exertion, 116
Physicians, 264–65; family stress and,
    24, 43, 58, 233; and medical informa-
    tion, 33–34, 101–2, 117, 121
Positive mental imaging, 231–32, 233
Precious Present (Johnson), 256
Price, Virginia, 164, 178, 179, 181
Procardia, 119
Progestin, 125

Psychological reactions, 8, 23, 142–43, 149–50, 158
Psychosomatic ailment, 55–56

Rahe, Richard, 229
Relaxation techniques, 113, 173, 206–7, 230–31, 232–33
Religion, 251
Reserpine, 119, 120
Rosenman, Ray, 160, 164, 212
Rosenthal, Saul, 118
Roskies, Ethel, 229

Satir, Virginia, 17, 48
Sedatives, 205, 227
Selective perception, 241
Self-esteem, 8, 29–30, 176, 178
Seligman, Martin, 247
Serpasil, 119
Sex over Forty (Rosenthal), 118
Sexual functioning, 78, 99, 128–33, 135–38; aging and, 104, 113, 122–26, 129, 131; and cardiovascular system, 115–17, 126–28, 138, 240–41; heart illness and, 100–102, 115, 116, 117, 127, 248; medication and, 117–21, 227; performance problems, 108, 109–14, 134; personality and, 133–34; sex drive, 102–7; sexual response cycle, 107–9, 123–24
Siegel, Bernie S., 226
Simonton, Carl, 233
Simonton, Stephanie, 233
Smoking, 37
Social support, 202, 234
Spectatoring, 129, 158
Spouses: in cardiac rehabilitation, 35, 77–78, 235; heart illness and, 25–26, 100, 154, 224–25; marriage stages and, 80, 81–82, 83–85; power struggles, 56–59; of Type A personalities, 162, 163, 168–70, 174–75, 183–86, 187, 189, 195, 197, 198, 200
Stimulants, 205, 227
Stress: balancing of commitments and, 225; and cardiac rehabilitation, 163, 238; disruption of family structure, 6–7, 12–13, 17–18, 47, 48–50, 52, 60; family overprotectiveness, 4,

189–90; healthy family coping, 16, 27, 29; illness as stressor, 8, 9–10, 11, 219–20; marital effects, 10, 11, 78, 252; medication and, 227–28; psychological reactions, 142–43, 144; sexual effects, 102, 107; and spouses of Type A personalities, 189–90, 191; thinking patterns and, 245–46; Type A reactions, 165, 170–72, 193–94, 208–9
Stress management, 3, 37, 207, 208–9, 226–36
Superperson state, 178–80, 182, 195
Surgery, 22–23; coronary bypass, 36, 42; penile, 126
Sympathetic blockers, 119–20

Tenormin, 119, 120
Testosterone, 104, 118, 124
Testosterone replacement therapy, 104
Therapists, 263–66
Thinking habits, 246, 247
Thought stopping, 211
Time management, 228
Trance-Formations (Grinder and Bandler), 231–32
Trandate, 119, 120
Transactional analysis, 143–44
Treadmill testing, 36, 116
Triangulation, 61–62, 63–64, 66–67, 69, 70–72
Type A personality, 134, 159; behavioral patterns, 58, 160–62, 164–67, 248; behavior change, 202–4, 212–16; and cardiac rehabilitation, 160, 162–64; environmental factors and, 207–9; heart illness risk, 161, 163, 165, 171–72, 202; hot reactors, 171–72, 173–75, 196, 203; and marital intimacy, 78, 162, 163, 197, 201, 248; marriage patterns, 186–201; physiology, 170–71, 203, 205–7; psychological development, 175–77; psychological states, 178–82, 195; spouses of, 162, 163, 168–70, 174–75, 183–86, 187, 189, 195, 197, 198, 200; stress reactions, 170–72; thinking pattern modification, 209–12

Type B personality, 198, 200; behavioral characteristics, 165, 170, 171, 172; heart patients, 162; spouses of Type A personalities, 162, 187–88, 195

Ulcers, 126
Ulmer, Diane, 164, 203, 204, 211, 212
Uterine cancer, 125

Vagina, 112, 124–25
Vaginismus, 112–13
Vaillant, George, 247
Vasodilators, 119, 120
Vasotec, 119

Wake Forest University Cardiac Rehabilitation Program, 14, 36

Weight, 120, 121
When Bad Things Happen to Good People (Kushner), 249
Williams, Redford, 164, 165, 211, 212, 215
Women: sexual problems, 111–13, 120, 124–25; sexual response cycle, 104, 107, 108, 109, 110; spouses of Type A personalities, 187, 188, 189–91; Type A personalities, 161, 177, 184–85
Work, 223–24, 225
Workaholics, 160

Zilbergeld, Bernie, 131

Heart Illness and Intimacy

Designed by Ann Walston

Composed by Brushwood Graphics, Inc.
in Meridien Medium with Meridien Bold Italic display

Printed by R. R. Donnelley & Sons Company
on 50-lb. S.D. Warren's Cream White Sebago,
and bound in Holliston Aqualite
with Simpson Evergreen end sheets.